2 in 1 to
Achieve Healthy well-Being

Acute or Chronic Pain in the Back,

Neck, Head, Sciatica, Shoulders?

Sciatica Exercises + Yoga for Pain Relief

Will Help You Solve Them

William M Wittmann

Table Of Contents

Sciatica Exercise

Simple Techniques, Stretching And Yoga Exercises To Find Relief From Back Pain And Sciatica. Recover Your Life Forever Without Drugs Or Surgery

William M Wittman

CHAPTER ONE

✑

Understanding sciatica

The definition of sciatica identifies outward symptoms originating out of the peripheral nerve, that's the huge nerve generated from several large nerves which branch away from every side of the low spinal column. The nerves proceed through the entire buttock area on each side and continue down the back of each leg. Below the knee, then the plantar nerve divides in to two branches which proceed the leg into the foot and ankle. However, many people today telephone outward symptoms any place in the leg, authentic thoracic symptoms happen at the buttock area and might stretch the back part of the thigh and back to the upper leg and feet. Broadly speaking, the further bloated the guts is, the farther the indicators will probably expand the leg down. When you'll find rare neurological disorders, which could cause the progression of sciatica as a result of lead nerve pathology, in the majority of cases sciatica can be really a symptom of several other underlying problem. Even the most prevalent causes of sciatica could be simplified in to two major categories, nerve wracking and muscular contraction. Nerve compression may be a consequence of various causes, however it's most frequently due to a bulge or insertion of a couple of intervertebral disks in the low thoracic spinal column.

Sciatica is pain at the back or hip that radiates on to the buttock and back of the leg across the sciatic nerve, usually to the foot. Each nerve transmits signals for motor controller of several muscles at the leg in addition to sensation towards the leg. The pain generated is resulting from an affected or inflamed gastrointestinal tract wracking and may appear after a personal accident, muscular stress, or herniated disc that presses on the guts.

Which exactly are the outward indicators?

The pain of sciatica usually takes quite a few forms - it can seem as a cramp in the leg, pain up on sitting, pain along with coughing or sneezing, and could arrive as tingling, tingling, burning, electric jolt such as sensation or as "pinsand needles" across the leg. The pain often occurs on a single side. Many individuals have sharp pain in 1 area of their hip or leg and numbness in different pieces. The senses might also be felt over the back of the calf or over the sole of their foot. Muscle fatigue may happen due to pressure or pain on the guts.

The pain often begins slowly and progressively becoming worse; definite activities can commence the observable symptoms for example;

Sitting or standing for extended intervals

At nighttime

When coughing, coughing, or laughing

When bending backward or walking than a couple of yards, particularly if due to spinal stenosis

Which exactly are the causes?

The sciatic nerves are the longest nerves in your system, running out of the lower back down the buttock and cool, and continuing down the back part of every leg entirely into the foot. Each carry neural signals for motor controller of several muscles from the leg in addition to sensation towards the leg.

Such a thing that combats a sciatic nerve for prolonged amounts of time could lead to sciatica. Sometimes this is caused by a ruptured disk in the low spine. In case the disk ruptures, their inner linking substance can float and shove against nerves. Age-related modifications to the backbone induce degeneration of these disks and also the vertebral tissues. Intervertebral discs make space between your bones, so allowing a location for those nerves to maneuver while they leave the back. Degeneration of these vertebrae may give rise to a narrowing of the distance between nerves which make a difference to a nerve root that induces similar signs.

Traumatization out of an auto crash or blow into the backbone may harm the sciatic nerve right away, because may muscle breeds of this lower back muscles and nerves of the piriformis muscle which runs directly across the guts. Since these muscles act as tight or move into anxiety, they are able to cause a rope-like strain which disturbs the nerve.

In addition to growing older, being at work which demands constant twisting, heavy lifting or forcing may make you likely to sciatica. The sitting which does occur as a consequence of a desk-job or being too sedentary may additionally put extra strain on the back and legs.

Evidence and tests

Sciatica may possibly be shown by way of a neurological and orthopedic study of their spine and thighs. Pain down the leg might be duplicated by lifting your leg straight off the table. Tests are guided by the suspected cause of this disorder, according to the history, symptoms, and pattern of symptom improvement.

Under ordinary conditions, there's loads of space around the spinal cord nerves by which they branch off from the back and then leave the spine (technically, the cervical back finishes at the middle thoracic spinal column and becomes a package of different nerves called the cauda equina at the low lumbers, however for the interest of simplicity, then i will be speaking about it since the back). However, the opening at which the nerve exits the spine may get substituted by a couple of stuff, leading to compression and irritation of the nerves. Probably one of the very typical sources of neural compression is that a disk bulge, that can also be referred to as a disk herniation, or disk protrusion. The disks have a outer cartilage wall and also are full of a gel-like material that offers the spine with numerous angles of freedom and shock-absorption. The wall may get damaged (in a sense which are going to probably be discussed later) and the inner pressure of the gel makes it bulge out at the tip of damage. On account of the arrangement of their spine, and owing to the activities and postures which we typically participate in, disks have a tendency to bulge backward towards the back and nerves.

The huge vast majority of disk injuries are emptied or protrusions and may usually be effectively treated with the strategy which may be discussed within this publication. Disc ruptures (extrusions) tend to be somewhat more severe and may frequently require operation to attain long-term aid of symptoms. Incidentally, the definition of "ruptured disc" usually gets used wrongly (by health practitioners) to explain what's obviously a disk bulge (herniation or protrusion), and thus do not assume you will require operation if you're told there is a ruptured disc and soon you've got confirmation (in an mri or ct scanning) that the disk remains actually pliable (the provisions "extruded" or "sequestered" may show up on the imaging accounts in reference to a couple of disks) and never merely bulging or protruding. Along with disk lumps and ruptures, the distance around the spinal nerves are usually narrowed by fluctuations inside the spine associated with rheumatoid arthritis. With rheumatoid arthritis, the disks may frequently eliminate fluid and eventually become slimmer, bone fractures can thicken or shape spurs, and spinal nerves can inhale (from the bones becoming closer together) or become thicker -- each one which might narrow down the openings that the nerves pass through.

To locate the treatment for sciatica you first need to begin understanding its own nature. This appears to be an extremely straightforward job but there several individuals who translate sciatica because of a easy straight back issue. But, it's different in contrast to a normal back ache. Sciatica is clarified to be a piercing kind of headache along with electric shocks and shocks. That really is by the inflammation which starts in the plantar nerve. The sciatic nerve is the major nerve which conducts sensory purposes by the decreased spine entirely down to the feet.

The function of the sciatic nerve from the body is very essential as it's in charge of relaying information to the mind.

It's accountable for organizing movement controller and sensory feedback of their feet and legs. There are lots of probable causes of the beginning of sciatica. The most prevalent disease is called a herniated spinal disk. The disk functions as a cushion into the back vertebra. But in the event the disk slides from its original location, it occupies the space for the nerves. Insulin begins, also sciatica develops. Other cases of illnesses that activate sciatica are piriformis syndrome and spinal stenosis.

The treatment for sciatica isn't exactly the exact same for several sufferers. Sciatica can be a symptom of an underlying origin. Step one towards a laughter treatment is discovering the particular condition. Consult a seasoned doctor regarding sciatica. Establishing a highly efficient cure will start with a full medical history test, accompanied closely by clinical exams such as an Xray. These evaluations are given only in the event the physician deems them to be mandatory.

To heal sciatica is always to cover the inflammation. Medical professionals urge simple bed rest and avoiding strenuous pursuits. Medicines for anti-inflammatory and muscular relaxing purposes tend to be prescribed to the individual. In acute cases of oral steroids for a much more competitive dose of anti-inflammation are also prescribed. Patients can also go for an epidural steroid injection. This can become an immediate anti remedy for sciatica. Some traditional sufferers of sciatica prefer ice and heat packs application to the bloated area to treat the pain.

Addressing the inflammation and pain are partial remedies of sciatica. Many caregivers encourage patients to run carefully constructed exercises mixed in using physical therapy sessions. This will assist in preventing future swelling episodes.

A surgical process for the treatment cure is most likely the last alternative for patients. In lots of instances, medical procedures is unnecessary. But, it ought to be seriously contemplated when puberty isn't treated after around a few weeks of subsequent nonsurgical cure approaches.

Sciatica operation intends in order to steer clear of compression, hence providing the regular distance for the thoracic nerve to work normally. The physician might want to clean a bone surrounding the guts or eliminate a broken disk. Luckily, a fantastic proportion of folks are wholly healed from sciatica without having to undergo operation. All these are the individuals whose plantar nerves aren't injured forever. Enough timeframe to treat pain will be in 3 months to a few months for a lot of cases. Sciatica at a mild or moderate form isn't regarded as a health emergency however also the distress and pain it attracts may disturb some body from living a regular living. Hence, the best choice is to look for the help of your physician once you've the earliest signs of sciatica and learn as far as possible regarding the treatment choices which are best for you personally.

Sciatica is an indication of an accident or disease that's affecting the plantar nerve at the leg. The sciatic nerve can be found from the decreased backbone throughout the thighs, also is a significant muscle for having the capability to maneuver and texture pieces of one's own leg, commanding all it. Sciatica is made up of pain, tingling, fatigue and also tingling at the leg. But these signs may fluctuate widely in many individuals.

Which exactly are the indicators of sciatica?

As said, sciatica could be experienced in a number of diverse ways. A few accounts that a pain that is dull, but some report mild numbness, or perhaps a burning pain. The pain is usually localized to a single side of their human body and the individual can experience it just 1 leg or one among her or his spine. These symptoms may worsen when standing up unexpectedly, at that nighttime, when vibration from laughing or alternative pursuits along with later long walks and physical exercise.

So, what can I really do concern sciatica?

Take part doing press ups, this will aim the principal nuisance are as within sciatica, the buttocks, the thighs and the spine side. Extension exercises are a more low-impact means to be certain you are perhaps not in pain after. For those who have use of some pool, then ask your personal doctor concerning water exercises, that is a excellent, painless approach to get started establishing your own strength. Hamstring exercises are fantastic for handling lower back pain.

Hamstring work-outs

There are some powerful exercises for strengthening your mind. Lying leg curls - it's called hamstring curl. You want to lie to your hamstring machine on tummy whilst setting the leg curl bar all on your knees. You want to launch it then repeat it to get a long time. Great mornings - you ought to set a barbell on your shoulders while keeping your legs inflexible at position. You want to bend forwards slightly, however, the mind ought to be upwards. You've got to create your torso parallel to the ground floor. Repeat it many times.

As a result of the disposition of sciatica, there may be an inherent problem which a health care provider should tackle. Exercise can be a superb solution to diminish painful senses and boost freedom. It's actually vital that you exercise to handle the pain, as it strengthens your muscles, providing more aid, and also perhaps not only does it reduce strain, it will also allow you to prevent it later on. You need to speak to your health care provider prior to getting involved in any strenuous training.

A variety of distress are advocated by a lady who's pregnant. The cause for this may be that the climbing weight that puts strain on the rear part and thighs. Few woman additionally undergo thoracic nerve pain throughout the time period. Occurrence with the could cause extreme debilitating from the normal uneasy disquiet. The sciatica nerve may be the largest nerve in your human body that stimulates and regulates the movement of their lesser portion of their human anatomy. Whenever there's swelling and compression found from the body, pressing activity pressures the thoracic nerve resulting in severe pain.

Women who complain of thoracic nerve pain that's sharp and popping the back part of the thighs, have undergone exactly the same before maternity. Some of the chief explanations for occurrence of this pain is protracted focusing in their toes and excess weight reduction. The perfect method to decrease the pain will be always to lay to among those negative. This specific posture lowers the total weight in the back along with your thighs. Depending on the character of tasks which can be performed in day to day existence, an individual has to set postures so. This measure reduces the maturation of sciatica and decreases the pain at the back and leg.

Sciatica nerve pain may be lowered by giving warmth into your system. Usage of hot compresses, a hot tub and also a restricted temperature at the room will avert the bitterness of annoyance. It's always recommended to not make use of heels throughout pregnancy since they induce discomfort and boost the degree of sciatica. Usage of comfortable shoes with soft feet is much more preferable since they feature nil or diminished stress growth in the foot. Routine exercises will reduce the quantity of stress developed from the low back section of the human anatomy.

It really is additionally crucial to seek advice from a health care provider for approval to perform certain exercises to avoid overtraining nerve pain. Swimming is among the most useful available exercises which stop the maturation of sciatica. Pregnant woman may also look forwards for rectal yoga which provides increased rest by the worries and increases the sum of relaxation. When the pain is more bothersome, an individual has to stop by a physical therapist who'll offer help by embracing special exercises which may enhance the potency from the elements of abdomen, spine and abdominal muscles. Sciatica occurs because of temporary disorder when pregnant and will be over come little preventative steps.

Where does the pain come out?

Sciatica anxiety is pain which elicits from the reduced part of their human body due to a issue with the peripheral nerve. Many times, that is from a lumbar disc herniation which moves down on the guts. But, pinched nerves, nerve wracking, inflammation, muscular issues, injuries, or germs may be the main reason.

Can be sciatica a significant problem?

Sometimes the pain which results in sciatica are able to keep people from contributing their lives for days and sometimes maybe weeks, also could be painful at a few cases.

Sciatic nerve issues may lead to pain, a sense of tingling, soothes tingles, and burning sensations at the reduced back off to the thigh. If the signs and symptoms are intense, they are able to interfere with the ability to walk or proceed at the midsection area. Anxiety relief for back pain can be potential, however it isn't just a challenge which may be mended immediately.

Can it be crucial to find a physician?

Should you suspect you have sciatic nerve difficulties, visit your personal doctor. He'll examine your health history and provide you with a detailed examination to establish what the issue is. Fixing the underlying problems could reduce recurrences of coronary artery pain. You may well be asked to get some evaluations such as for example x-rays, MRI scans, and scans, or even electromyogram. Don't try to diagnose or cure yourself. *

So, what exactly can be done to halt the pain?

From the ago, bedrest has been certainly one of the principal treatments for sciatica. Recent studies demonstrate that bed rest is really not the most suitable choice. Bed remainder prevents you out of proceeding, and movement is obviously valuable. Various other kinds of therapy that can help with pain relief and reduce inflammation may be· exercising by extending

Your doctor may provide you a set of pain-relieving stretching. Once the pain has improved, in case you carry on using those stretches, then they are able to cut the odds of pain killers at the foreseeable future. Strengthening muscles to boost your posture can be a fantastic means to decrease the prospect of gastric pain coming back again.

Surgical processes

There are distinct kinds of operation which may help alleviate gastrointestinal pain. But, operation is a really aggressive treatment that's most frequently utilized in chronic scenarios.

Infection direction

Infection management experts will assist you to handle continuing pain difficulties. These professionals make use of various techniques depending on the intensity of one's situation. Treatment may involve medication, physical therapy or topical software or emotional therapy.

in case you believe you're experiencing the signs and symptoms of sciatic nerve pain, so you need to contact your primary care doctor when you can explore all your treatment choices.

Every person differs therefore every individual's treatment plans will probably differ. Chronic pain is never a standard condition. There are tons of options outside there which may assist you in getting on with a balanced and regular daily life.

CHAPTER TWO

❦

Degenerative bone and ligament thickening

Degenerative changes from the backbone most frequently influence the trunk portion of their spinal openings, whilst disk lumps and ruptures usually narrow front of their spinal pockets. Oftentimes, there's a level of narrowing from the disk protrusion and degenerative alterations. Additionally, further nerve wracking frequently results in swelling as a result of inflammation that's set off by disk damage or degenerative arthritis. While nerve wracking may also lead from spinal and pancreatic ailments that require operative therapy, the vast majority of instances of nerve wracking are caused by a mix of disk bulging, degenerative alterations, or inflammatory swelling and may usually be efficiently handled with the remedies mentioned in this publication. The other big group of reasons for sciatica symptoms is muscular contraction. Several muscles could lead to pain down the leg but merely a single muscle really meets the indicators of authentic sciatic nerve distress. The piriformis is a muscle situated in the low buttock area on each side which attaches out of the sacrum (the triangular bone at the bottom of their spine) into the top femur, just below the hip joint.

Anatomy of this spine

A summary of the spine

The spine can be a intricate portion of one's entire body, also will be divided up to three major categories. The backbone comprises the bones which make up your backbone, such as the disks. Secondly there are neurological elements in the spinal column, like the spinal cord and nerve roots. The remaining weather of one's backbone can also be categorized as encouraging structures. These structures comprise muscles, ligaments, joints, and ligaments.

The backbone

We will center on the backbone, and this is composed of the selection of bones present on your spine, where the ribs hook up with. The spinal column serves lots of functions and purposes. When it comes to its purpose from the spine, it gives a base for attachment of both their backbone ligaments, bones, tendons, and joints. It protects the spinal cord, nerve roots, and lots of organs, and provides the major structural aid for nearly all of one's entire body, as well as the chest, shoulders, and torso. The spine gives the system proper balance and weight reduction, in addition to allows your chest to own the variety of motion it will, such as bending forwards, backward, laterally, and also rotate.

Anatomy

The spinal column is composed of both 32-34 individual nerves, which are the bones that give the cornerstone for the spinal column. These bottoms are broken up into five major categories, depending on their position on the spinal column. Starting at the bottom of the skull, then you will find seven cervical vertebrae that comprise the neck. Below those we find 12 thoracic vertebrae, found in the top rear. The decrease spine (below the curve) includes 5 nerves called cervical nerves. Located only below those, there's a set of 5 vertebrae. All these are combined, or fused with each other to generate the sacrum, that's part of the pelvis. At the lower end of this backbone is that your coccyx, or tailbone. That really is created from 3 5 fused vertebrae.

Each human vertebra is composed of several components and each has exceptional features based on the area in that it can be available. Every vertebra, no matter position, has three basic operational parts: the drum-shaped body, designed to keep weight and defy loading or compression; the anterior (back side) arch, manufactured from this lamina, pedicles and facet joints; and also, the transverse procedures, to which muscles attach.

Between every one of those pliers are intervertebral disks, usually abbreviated to only "disks". All these are constructed from quite good, hard cells which relate each vertebra into another location. They have been in the leading part of the spine and so are what provide the chest the skill to go forward, backward, laterally, and also to rotate.

Minor body injuries are a recognized fact of life for anybody who contributes a relatively busy life style. However, if pain gets debatable and chronic, it can be the time to consult with professionals concerning exactly what may possibly be the foundation of this pain. A pinched nerve can be regarded as to blame in terms of chronic pain, particularly when it develops to spine pain, neck pain, leg pain, shoulder pain or hip pain. A chiropractor might be the solution for pain relief in this circumstance, and we'll explain how to establish whether that condition may possibly be at the origin cause of one's pain.

Infection

The expression pinched nerve can be employed in medicine to explain a injury or harm to a single nerve or pair of nerves for almost any variety of explanations. The nerve mostly influenced by this affliction is that the sciatic nerve-wracking, also as it's bundles which encircle through the entire human body, it might lead to pain in are as far removed from the true injury website. As a result of the, in case you reveal the following symptoms, it could have been a smart idea to visit your regular doctor or physician instantly, so the trauma site might be ascertained, and therapy began.

Weakness: generally sensed in a extremity, such as, for instance, a leg or arm, but might usually pose itself at the back too. Is such as the muscles positioned in that field are tremendously feeble, and might lack standard strength whilst controlling them.

Tenderness: your skin, tendons and muscle inside the affected area are vulnerable to observable feelings, such as anxiety, pain, compression and extension. The complete area around the affected nerve package feels sore, such as it'd experienced acute discomfort during a very long time period.

Odd sensations: you could feel strange sensations in the affected spot, such as hooks and needles, tingling and waves of burning sensations or traumatic and changing pains. These can also coincide with muscular aches, and therefore are caused by the compression or portion of those neural bundles.

Reasons

The principal reason behind this affliction can be straightforward effort. As soon as we work hard or play hard, we run the chance of pulling muscles straining joints, and changing a number of our fragile bones out of place, particularly as we grow old. Age can be a variable for the 2nd almost certainly cause of the illness, that will be bone marrow or thickening of their bones during arthritis and aging. This may be quite a defining variable for the precise location of this compression, specially once the sciatic nerve is included.

Additional medical conditions, such as sciatica, herniated disks, and spinal stenosis could create the nerve packs across the backbone to become compacted, literally pinching the lymph vessels and also causing pain to radiate all through the human anatomy. This is the reason it's essential to be analyzed to find out the origin of the compression or injury. Too frequently the website is supposed to be at which the pain is, even if the truth is, it could be far removed as a result. Last, any injury which includes the neck, knee, spine or back may cause the vertebrae which form the spine to compress or shift, and also the spinal nerves combined with it.

Treatment options

The treatment with this illness is normally broken into stages of treatment choices. For chronic pain episodes, treatment with corticosteroid shots, accompanied by periods of bedrest, will probably alleviate the many debilitating symptoms. Chiropractic adjustments may be performed, in addition to physical therapy sessions. The trick to any workable treatment program, nevertheless, is examinations and assessments to nail the wounded location.

Can you realize that chronic pain signals traveling throughout your system quicker compared to sensory signature signs? It will and that's the reason why so many men and women use massage as an adjunct for their own pain control regimen. Ostensibly the therapists signature starts together with all the chronic pain signals traveling through the back (because this may be the pathway for several nerve-conduction) and signature wins every moment! While this could well not indicate no annoyance for you personally, it's going to absolutely mean less pain through the whole period of your massage and regularly for a time period afterward. Twist even competes with severe pain signs:(think: stub your toe) and that's the reason we instinctively reach to our hurt dig-it and hold it before the pain diminishes. Or mothers kiss a booboo. The signature signal goes faster. Regrettably the fee of massage could also be prohibitive for a great deal of individuals. 1 way to go around this would be to locate a massage school near. You may usually get an excellent massage to get a small percentage of the fee supplied by students who's over seen by an instructor. Then of course, there's always the choice of requesting a buddy or spouse to get a massage. Should you go that path you might want to get well prepared and also have some massage so that their hands will slide correctly. Nothing worse than having skin peeled from inadequate lotion or oil.

Along with while we are on the topic of chronic pain, have you noticed how stressed your muscles get when struck by an arctic burst? Our stance affects as we walk hunched over wanting to safeguard ourselves out of sub-par. If we need to stick out from sunlight for any amount of time we start to shiver, frequently with cable stressed muscles. That which can add up to is pain free in the future as we thaw out. The best remedy is prevention, so putting relaxation before fashion. I am constantly astonished at how my mature kids will groom their small ones into the hilt at the cold, however frequently wear just a fleece themselves. They laugh at me once i wear two kinds of trousers and a set of tights along with also my ill bean coat that's fantastic for 40 below after i move walking throughout subzero temperatures however, I actually don't care. I understand that layers are things keeps you warm and feel me coating such as mad! Therefore, that the next time you end up rubbing your shoulders and wondering just how they have so tender, inquire how hot you might be once you go out. The solution might surprise you.

Anatomy for fitness professionals

How to master muscular anatomy quick & prevent the 5 most shared anatomy mistakes

Anatomy = foundation of exercise science

Learning human anatomy for an exercise pro is similar to learning how to create a base being a architect; it affirms all else!

Everything else is constructed on top of it!

Personal training is very lively and romantic, therefore that i guess that you might make the exact same claim regarding personality being ; in case the client does not want to invest some time together with you as your lousy attitude or awful communication competencies, it really does not matter how far you realize!

However, that is the reason the reason why we split fitness sills in to categories. As training is indeed lively, it's effective to divide a variety of skillsets in to 3 important mega-competencies: social abilities and exercise science, and business acumen.

Anatomy and bio mechanics would be the foundation of practice science, together with physiology supplementary. (what's structure any way, except the anatomies answer to forces/mechanics? Don't hesitate to disagree from the comments, i understand that is simply not a favorite view, but i think that it really is worth analyzing)

Additionally, it doesn't matter just how far you understand about different regions of exercise science, even if you have a strong base in biomechanics and body, you won't have the capacity to safely and correctly employ your comprehension.

Different types of anatomy

Within body, you can find various targets; neural body, bony body, and muscular body. Like a trainer, it's vital to bear in mind just how a number of different structures there have been from your system which affects its operation and wellness.

Yes, initially we ought to really be centered on muscle body, however as caregivers, we must bear in mind we have a tendency to be overly dedicated to muscles some times. Many times, a tight muscle tends to tighten due to a fascial limitation! Everything is connected to all during the fascial network. Simply bear this in your mind whenever your trouble solving and analyzing.

As you progress, additional hours ought to be used learning heightened anatomy such as fascial body, and also the body of their joints, ligaments, tendons and also the way in which they connect to embryonic surfaces.

Exercise makes perfect

There is a great deal of great programs available to find body. Take advantage of these tools, the initial one is totally free, and exercise together with different coaches. Produce purchases quiz one another, and attempt to join the particular names to your exercise routine once you work out.

[anatomy for fitness] getbodysmart.com - this site is wonderful! It's an electronic digital cartoon of this muscle system. Drag on and drag just a tiny slider under each combined, and it'll construct the muscle support system round it by the deep into the superficial. Very cool and worth looking into, you may even click to observe each muscles activity, that will be good but very simplified. (make sure you browse "most frequent anatomy mistakes" below). And it's really completely free! Additionally, you will consider a quiz on the website. Every fresh fitness pro ought to know concerning this website and spending some time about it, it's good.

Person anatomy atlas of human body DVD set -this DVD collection is remarkable! I've observed all of those DVDS (the 6th one is all in regards to the organs). As soon as it's on the other side to find all 6 simultaneously, it's a excellent reference for anybody who would like to carry their own body into the second level. They ostensibly build an original cadaver facing you, together with precise animation to demonstrate each source and insertion. They begin with the rectal body, then build the muscles in deep to shallow at the top, reveal the cells from 360 viewpoints. They then reveal the neural and circulatory system, and also have connections involving each section. You might even begin with only 1 DVD at the same time, also watch only 10 minutes every day. It's fascinating! These complicated structures would be the bodies evolutionary reaction to force! DVD 1, 2, and 3 would be important for newer coaches, because they truly are upper extremity, lower extremity, and trunk/core.

Fitness anatomy strength training anatomy book - that is a superb publication. Step by step, vibrant, and just plain interesting to check at. The muscles examples have become much of a jacked human body builder, so it's maybe not exactly what you should normally find at a typical public client, however it's an awesome guide to basic human anatomy. There's perhaps not quite as much awareness to human anatomy of those "passive structures" (bones, tendons, ligaments) and spinal body.

Cadaver course - among the greatest ways to learn would be to really get your fingers dirty! I moved for the class and it was wonderful! We're so utilized to considering these cells as different, since they come in novels, however they're all merged together! This was eye opening to find the fibers of this rhomboid fan in to the fibers of this serratus! It looked just like one-muscle! Here is a URL into the site. They've a cadaver course in Pittsburgh and at Connecticut. If you're in yet another region of the earth, also you ought to have the ability to discover a cadaver class at any given university using courses that are related. The cool thing about the body optional is you're able to get continuing education credits, also it's a dependence on the resistance training professional certificate. But do not allow it to prevent you when you're not at or even Pittsburgh, look for a class and get the hands dirty!

Many common anatomiesmistake!

All these would be the largest mistakes which gym professionals and books create about body:

1. Inch. The activity of this muscular tissues is entirely determined by its own position! Yes your hip adductors move your thighs toward one another when they're abducted, but they'll expand the fashionable in the event that you're in the fashionable is fully flexed, or stretch the fashionable if it's fully flexed. If you're only beginning, aren't getting confused, simply concentrate on the obvious muscle activity, but bear in your mind that every muscles work is positional, also certainly will fluctuate dependent on the job of the joints.

2. Each muscle has some type of role in most single plane, and it's an outrageous activity, concentric activity, and isometric activity. Oh, also from every plane, " i really don't mean all of 3 airplanes since there's definitely an infinite number of airplanes (still another major yet common body mistake) what plane is cutting on out a barbell together with your own arm? In case that blows off your mind, i suggest choosing the rts certificate asap!

3. We often concentrate on shallow muscles and rectal muscles since they're easier to find and promote their dressing table! Don't make this mistake with your body or your own customers; without even equilibrium, equilibrium, and also the deeper/smaller stabilizers, you will wind up a cripple earlier or later!

4. Do perhaps not make an effort to impress your customers with your understanding of body! Naming the profound 6 trendy rotators won't impress your potential! Unless they're

a physician, then they'll just be confounded and perhaps insulting! Always confer with a client in a language that they know; that really is best for communicating and earnings. Yes, even while you create a partnership, you should enlarge your customer's knowledge in order that they simply take charge of these fitness, but then, focus going for technical comprehension and maybe not domains. At first, whenever they state "I need bigger arms, then they still seem to be older lady arms", you say"this app may specifically target people granny arms" you may sell more bundles ensured.

5. One other quick notice on speech. In all costs, avoid using the term "functional" where you ever would like simply to appear knowledgeable. Yes people want it, also it's a buzzword, however, keywords are frequently quite inefficient at communicating. Rather than "functional" state "workout or app x y z may allow you to work better in abc or function at abc or even move to activity abc". Major pet peeve of mine! Do not only sound smart when you're smart!

CHAPTER THREE

❦

Discovering the cause of your sciatica

Infection relief for sciatica pain can be actually a must, since the pain in the bloated or injured backbone guts might be so powerful it's completely painful. The sciatic nerve is the longest nerve in the body, running in the thoracic (smallest) region of the spine from the back in to the buttocks and down the thighs. Sciatica is a disorder brought on by irritation or pressure on that nerve which travels down its length, also along with pain, it can manifest itself like being a tingling, and a weakness, or even perhaps a tingling in the affected areas.

What exactly is the spine?

The spine is a loadbearing structure comprised of twenty-five construction blocks, called vertebrae. Each vertebra is simply a couple inches wide and nearly round in look. Additionally, it features a rounded hole close to the trunk, and also the holes out of every one of the vertebrae lineups perfectly to make the backbone. Nerves from the mind operate through the backbone and then down into the rest of the entire body.

In between your vertebrae are twenty-three disks, and each roughly one quarter of a inch thick. They function as shock absorbers and cushion the bones' little movement once your human body moves. The disks, unlike the fascia, aren't composed of bone rather they truly are a material like the ribs which creates your own nose. Sciatica may be the affliction which happens once the lumbar 4 5 disk (the disk between your fifth and fourth cervical vertebrae) irritates or puts pressure on the plantar nerve developing from the backbone.

What's sciatica pain treated?

Sciatica anxiety might be treated with numerous different conventional or other modalities, like those below.

Drug

Many cases of sciatica are treated with painkillers. In very mild conditions, the primary choice is over-the-counter remedies, such as ibuprofen, acetaminophen, aspirin, or naproxen. These may help decrease the pain and commence to correct tissue at precisely the exact same moment. They're all generally regarded as safe for momentary usage of healthy adults, however you shouldn't require them for two or more weeks at one time. You also need to not have some medications containing exactly the exact same active ingredients, since you may possibly harm your liver or other organs

Exercise

Exercise is your ideal method to decrease sciatica symptoms to the very long run. By training your muscles to develop into both strong and relaxed, it's going to help cut the total amount of pressure they employ into the thoracic nerve which runs throughout them. In the event the foundation of puberty is pressure out of the short, tight piriformis muscle, the muscle has to have been softly stretched. In the event the foundation of sciatica is by the bulging disk, gentle low spine strengthening and stretching exercises can help. Yoga moves can assist with source.

Workout is your reclined spinal spin. Utilize the following directions:

1. Inch. Lie flat on your back to a mat.
2. B ring up your knees to your chest, as close as possible
3. Stretch your arms to each side along with your palms down
4. Stick to the count of three.
5. Exhale into the use of five and also lower your knees slowly to the proper.
6. Sit and again bring back your knees into your own torso.
7. Exhale yet again, and also this time around lower your knees to your left side.
8. Come back into the center .
9. Repeat the exercise 8 10 times.

Earlier you start this or another workout routine, get hold of your physician or therapist to ascertain which exercises are ideal for you personally.

Alternative therapies

Fixing laughter might prove easier for several people using alternative as opposed to conventional treatments. Even though nontraditional therapies ordinarily would not need scientific proof of their advantages and security, lots of men and women find these helpful, in particular people individuals who have had no success with conventional measures.

Certainly, one of the most typical alternative remedies is chiropractic attention. Chiropractors cannot prescribe drugs, choose blood, nor do some invasive procedures, like a physician may; nevertheless, they ought to have a health history and complete physical exam, and, if justified, they could order diagnostic tests, like XRAYS and cat tests, and to decide whether there's a issue with the plantar nerve.

Chiropractors heal the full human body, together with the backbone because their specialization, and also the essence in their spinal modification therapy is dependent upon the specific reason for the sciatica. The health care provider will normally press your back to relieve swollen nerves and also boost movement on your joints. If the issue comes from a disk problem, the chiropractic way of is to alleviate anxiety to alleviate pain and restore much better motion to the spinal column joint.

Surgery

When all alternatives have failed, a physician may elect to carry out spinal operation. When herniated disks are the reason for sciatica pain, the physician may suggest doing a microdiscectomy, an operation which permanently eliminates anything is squeezing the nerve. Or, they may elect to get a discectomy, a procedure which involves removing the disk causing the issue, or the one that's laborious, in the spinal column. Once the disk was taken away, the pressure in the nerve is relieved and sciatica symptoms and pain are not reduced.

Together with treatment from sciatica, an individual has to additionally pay attention to the status which ends in the annoyance. There are lots of techniques of getting treatment from sciatica.

Sciatica causes horrendous back pain, as a result of pressure on the sciatic nerve. Sitting or standing for a protracted period or actions like biking for as long may also lead to sciatica. The damaging spreads out of the back into the buttocks and also to the foot.

To commence with, medications like aspirin, Tylenol and aspirin are normal to cut back both swelling and will also be known to decrease pain. Medicines should be obtained after a physician's management.

Second, besides medications, routine exercises may also be invaluable in providing pain relief in sciatica. In the event there is acute pain that a couple of days of bed rest might help in relieving the discomfort but also much bedrest has a negative effect. It disturbs the muscles and as an alternative of reducing pain an individual can wind off with further pain.

Thirdly, stretching exercises and massage treatments treat muscular aches and assist in preventing pain relief from your esophagus. Muscle migraines when left untreated; often to alleviate the suffering.

Fourthly, a proper sitting position is essential to reducing the strain also to protect against an excessive amount of stress about the back. Soft mattresses or jazzy seats utilized for sitting may create worse that the illness and build a hindrance from the method of cure.

Additional compared to the people cited, averting lifting heavy objects, cold and hot compressions, several all-natural treatments for example consuming raw garlic, garlic milk, olive oil, a balanced and nutritious diet containing vitamin b 1 improved vegetables and fruits, correct intake of drinking water and a couple things that you ought to follow to treatment from sciatica.

Should you have problems with the diminished back burning pain, so it could seem as though the pain actually melts, or melts down your leg again. That is frequently connected with pain. Sometimes, individuals who have sciatica may not suffer with some true pain in their spine, but many others have problems with acute pain. For those who are afflicted with this illness that commonly causes it to feel like though your spine, leg and on occasion the medial side of one's foot is on fire, then you aren't alone, because tens of thousands of people like you have problems from this illness. Actually, it's a lot more prevalent than you may think.

Certainly, one of the best means to begin curing your spine would be to identify what's causing your pain. For a few, this could be as easy as carrying a measure erroneously and others it might possibly be something. Many men and women who suffer with burning off back pain, report which it simply happens once they go their legs into the other side, or perform tasks that want parts of these own bodies to maneuver in an unusual angle. Whenever you will find exactly what it is that creates your own spine pain to wake up, you then certainly can modify your moves in a means which won't enable one to inflame your esophagus.

Most individuals who suffer with burning lower back pain may find respite from their pain by avoiding activities that activate the debilitating reaction, but many more aren't pleased to stop performing certain things indefinitely, and those are the men and women who decided they are finished with pain drugs and being made to sit to facilitate their back pain. They will work to locate a means to permanently cure back pain.

In case this sounds just as if you then you definitely need to be aware that recent studies have unearthed your burning lower back pain could be caused by a misalignment on the human physique. To put it differently, you have any muscles which are stronger than some others. At these times, the muscles always tug each other and induce the human body to become misaligned. Which usually means that more than the poorer muscles provide up and also the stronger ones may possibly be yanking your spine to an alternative position as it should naturally function inside. For a few, the muscles are often balanced in strength till they engage in something they're not utilized to, that'll subsequently pull on the spine out of alignment and cause the burning off lower back pain that lots folks identify as sciatica.

You are able to reduce and permanently expel burning off back pain by figuring out how to offer either side of one's own body equal potency. Whether you are interested in creating a area, like the shoulders stronger and more balanced, or would like to fortify the whole spine so you are strong completely round, you're able to discover how to safely and efficiently balance your own body so you can eliminate the burning off back pain that you have problems with without pain drugs of any sort.

Just how can you know that you're having gastrointestinal nerve pain? You might feel pain on your back and also that pain will start to radiate on your buttocks and can gradually get into a own leg again. In the event you're feeling are undergoing such a pain, then you may possibly be experiencing sciatica.

Sciatica is a disorder that affects thousands of people in

the whole world. From the west that it accounts for more than 80 per cent of the mature people's backpain issues. At the USA of America, over 7.5 million adults suffer with alcoholism as well as this illness is the reason its 2nd most prevalent reason people see their health practitioners each day.

The causes with the pain vary however, probably the most common of them include; a pinched sciatic nerve induced by the inflammation of the nearby joints; spinal disk herniation due to improper posture or consequent in wrongly damaging your spinal column disk whilst reaching out for something; there's yet another cause called this piriformis syndrome - that the piriformis may be that the muscle located in the buttocks; sciatica may be caused by spinal stenosis or ovarian cysts.

This informative article can look at methods by that you'll be able to find the relief you're looking for the pain. If you browse on till the conclusion, you are going to see an easy method to obtain invaluable advice relating to this illness that'll make certain you don't need to suffer out of this again on your own life. Countless people in more than 93 countries of the world used this way to treat their sciatica forever.

You are able to get relief for the own pain without even choosing for operation since a lot of individuals do. (as a primary alternative for this matter, do you think it?) Deciding on operation when you will find noninvasive operative methods to this predicament is mad. (would not you agree?)

The most common sciatic pain alleviation is choosing for maids or non-steroidal anti-inflammatory drugs. All these are all over the counter medications that help bring relief into parts of your muscles.

Subsequently there's also physical therapy including low impact exercise patterns such as; swimming, rowing, yoga, Taiichi, walking, extending and so forth. All these have the additional benefit of one's having the ability to do them in home.

Additional techniques that you may possibly like to take to are the next; massage-therapy, the usage of heat and ice packs, chiropractic methods, homeopathic treatments, the usage of blossoms and so forth.

Relieving symptoms with ice and heat

Among the ordinary confusion's folks have with self-treatment could be your matter of when to make use of ice cream and when to make use of heat. Once we discussed in the prior phase, ice hockey is more preferable once the matter is just one of nerve wracking, whilst heating is significantly better for sciatica because of muscular regeneration. In the previous chapter we discussed several hints about ascertaining the reason for one's symptoms, however if in doubt, a very simple guideline is always to base your choice of whether to use heat or ice on precisely what the signs are. When you've got intense or sharp pain without swelling, then this typically implies there was inflammation gift, also this can be a opportunity to make use of ice cream. On the flip side, if your symptoms are for the most part mild or stiffness annoyance, there's not often substantial inflammation present, also this circumstance, heat can be a much greater choice. As a precaution, unless you've undergone a trauma, or think it's likely you have injured yourself, it's ideal to refrain from heat for at least 4-8 hours to be certain the inflammatory response will not be triggered and the redness has not had enough time to install. When in doubt, stay clear of heat! Even though heat might feel well although it's on (because heat increases transmission of certain neural signals which hurt signs to be somewhat obstructed by achieving the brain), heat increases the inflammatory response to the human anatomy. Increased inflammation means raised pain whenever you quit using heat. Even though ice might well not seem too comfortable as heating, it really is among the very best anti-inflammatory measures you may take. The temporary disquiet of employing ice usually pays in long-term aid. Even though some experts recommend alternating heat and ice (as an instance, 10 minutes of ice hockey accompanied by 10 minutes of heat), i haven't seen any specific advantage by this way. In most cases, choosing one or another predicated on the outward symptoms as was only discussed is usually the easiest way and within my own experience works only as well or better than wanting to substitute the remedies. No matter whether you're employing heat or ice, you always need to divide the hot or ice bunch out of skin using a coating of fabric to reduce skin damage. It's likewise essential to avoid using heat or ice on a place that's been treated with, icy hot, bio freeze, ben-gay, or even any further topical ointment - wait before impression of this analgesic has worn away, otherwise the heat or ice can lead to skin damage or annoyance. Additionally, when utilizing either heat or ice, you should only use the procedure for approximately 1-5 minutes at one time, allowing your skin to return to normalcy temperature (to be safe and allow 1 or 2 hours) prior to applying the treatment. Because it could have a couple of minutes to your cold or hot sensation to produce it through the cloth layer between your cold/hot pack as well as skin, start time when you begin to feel that the temperature shift on the epidermis area.

Crucial note*: if you've got diminished flow or diminished skin sensitivity because of nerve injury, diabetes, etc., and it's ideal to consult with your health care provider first before employing heat or ice.

Sciatica symptom relief exercises

There are various exercises which were indicated for its self-treatment of sciatica. I frequently encounter individuals who've been awarded long, complicated lists of exercises by either doctors or physical therapists. The majority of those exercises are of nominal benefit in the optimal and on account of the intricacy of the physical exercise regime, many patients do not utilize them to get long-term. In my 20 plus years of clinical experience have discovered that using a few especially effective exercises to an average basis is a lot more beneficial than just having patients perform a whole lot of unique exercises. Within this phase, i will be introducing exercise tips which are designed to relieve pain as fast as achievable. While major ailments are found, i recommend that an "intensive care" way into the exercises at which frequent reproduction is the trick to symptom relief. The idea of copying is just one which i do wish to highlight because I've given these tips to tens of thousands of people through the past few years throughout my chiropractic office in addition to my blogs and online instructional videos and also the requirement for frequent reproduction in early phases of treatment is always missed. That is probably simply because of the manner that exercises are normally exhibited by health practitioners and physicians. The typical manner that exercises for sciatica have been exhibited is the affected individual has been led by them at a physician's or therapist's office at a supervised treatment session lasting 15 to 30 minutes together with treatment sessions daily or another day, or so the patient is only supplied a sheet of exercises and also told to complete them in your home. In the beginning, together with all these procedures, the patient does the exercises one or two times every day. For neural compression sciatica linked to a bulging disc, which is inadequate to acquire lasting relief speedily, therefore patients may frequently select all weeks or months in pain using very slow advancement.

Today you might be convinced that is clearly a lot - and it's also, but the majority of individuals won't need to maintain up this frequency for long. Typically, a couple days into a couple weeks of multiple times a hour utilization of those exercises i am going to show will radically lower the symptoms, so when this does occur, you're able to decrease the frequency of these exercises into merely several minutes daily to avoidance (as we'll discuss in the chapter about prevention and rehab). The particular frequency of these exercises may vary significantly in line with this individual. As a rule of thumb, for individuals up to approximately 50 decades old, it is suggested starting with doing each exercise for about one minute at one time in a frequency of 5 to 6 days daily. For folks over 50, i would recommend you start with a frequency of roughly 50% that at two to three times each day. That is only because elderly individuals frequently have a certain amount of arthritis, which is temporarily annoyed by the indicated exercises. Lots of men and women would find some good discomfort inside their shoulders or backs throughout the "intensive maintenance" period of their exercises. That may be temporary, and may typically be eased with using ice as discussed earlier in the day, and/or using massage. Provided that the soreness is still tolerable, i suggest continuing with all the exercises at the recommended frequency, however you always have the option to lessen the frequency of this exercise if needed. 1 final point of clarification before i move in to the exercises will be that the simple fact from the perspective of the overall health of nerves, numbness is much worse than annoyance. Even though the majority of men and women notice numbness to become comfortable compared to pain, tingling indicates longer or greater interval nerve compression compared to pain really does. Consequently, if you're beginning mostly together with numbness also it really is shifting to pain, then that's in fact a fantastic sign ordinarily. On the flip side, should you begin with mostly pain and it's shifting to numbness, that's often a poor sign and is still an indicator you need to change what you're doing or find professional therapy. That said it's crucial to tell apart numbness, and it is a deficiency of sense, from "heaviness" or"fatigue" that sometimes does occur for a brief period after acute pain goes off. If you are uncertain that you're having, gently jab the effected area having a needle or pin (that you really don't have to break skin) and compare the impression to the very same area across the other side of one's own body or yet another area that feels ordinary and also compare them. In case the pin/needle feels roughly the exact same on either areas, you're most likely simply experiencing heaviness leading to muscles relaxing since the neural soreness diminishes.

Mckenzie procedure (called for physical therapist robin McKenzie) are frequently related to expansion (backward bending) of their spine, in reality they're about analyzing, after which exercising, stretches and positions which facilitate or produce "centralization" of outward symptoms. Centralization signifies that the outward symptoms proceed nearer into the spinal column. As an instance, when you've got low back pain with sciatica (leg pain), then centralization are at which in fact the observable symptoms leave or decrease at the leg, then even when pain remains the exact same or gets worse at the buttocks or even low back again.

Perhaps you are aware about prostate massage and you're wondering why "how i could utilize prostate massage that will help my climax?" well, this sensual massage may truly be a enormous assistance give your guy a trackable discharge. However, "just how would you do precisely that?" I've got the solution for both questions.

You can utilize the prostate massage as a way to present your man an alternative sort of orgasm. It's a discharge that could be tremendously intense when compared with the customary orgasm he's. Some men that have tried this strategy assert this is the man variation of multiple climaxes. If done correctly with caution, the bliss will absolutely follow along with

If you're prepared to assist your person attain prostate orgasm, then you must prepare yourself with the odd procedure of researching the interiors of the anus. Don't stress. There's a suitable means that you safely perform so massage. You don't need to feel afraid that you may damage your individual. Provided that you follow my hints, you are just going to be fine.

First thing you need to accomplish is to speak to your

partner with regards to your sake of wanting this particular massage. You can not only surprise him as this may possibly hamper the catastrophic effect of this experience. It took me my fan sometime until we successfully reached vaginal climax. It needs a considerable quantity of time and a great deal of patience.

Some of the first problems you need to manage will be the positioning. You will kneel before your partner while he's standing. Take your hands between his thighs, and hit out because of his butt with your hands before you personally. When he fails to feel more comfortable with this particular position, you might just ask him to lie on his back and then open his or her legs. Within this position you can easily get his prostate and penis.

You're absolutely free to detect different places that could do the job with you both. I recommend you don't rush to converse in your own very first effort. Only go slow. Start with being comfortable with only touching his ass. You will touch his manhood as you're researching his anal area. This will be quite gratifying for him personally.

It's not exactly about the massage and also the processes. It's also wise to let your fan believe that you're appreciating the sight, so that you like what you're doing. This are the ideal turnon for the partner. When he sees that you also receive pleasure from pleasing himhe would be happy. Thus, make eye contact and speak with him as you're carrying out these.

All these are the necessities that you might want once you try so prostate massage: caliber paper and paper towels. The lubricant will assist you along with your partner using penetration. You really do want decent lubricant at there because his anal area isn't utilized for the sort of sensation. To help relieve his muscles and also to produce the penetration smooth, then the lubricant may help you.

Paper towels are for the litter you may possibly create. With the typical orgasm, the consequences of this discharge is a lot thinner. Inside this massage, the semen will be watery and also the total amount will be greater. That is a result of the fluid out of his prostate. Thus, prepare yourself with a paper towels which means that you might prevent the mess.

Proceed and research with your own man. I promise you he is going to be pleased with the prostate massage you'll likely be providing him. At this time, you're already targeted with the suitable knowledge that'll permit one to employ prostate massage that will assist you to man orgasm.

Even as we grow old are muscles and tendons become stiffer. For lots of individuals their own bodies also have undergone multiple cycles of trauma, inflammation and pain, some level of reimbursement in the region of trauma, and version of their surrounding tissues, ligaments and tendons. Once the redness subsides as well as the pain has been eliminated, either from medications or rest, they believe that they have been treated. Regrettably, these injuries frequently lead to misaligned joints which don't go as well and muscular adhesions causing decreased endurance. Your system will adaptively go on to prevent pain throughout this episode. Based upon the length of pain and the quantity of structures required a specific level of reimbursement does occur. All this results on your own body changing how it moves and conveys it self.

In otherworld's movement routines vary now follow the

course of least resistance. With the years the quantity of muscle fibers ready for movement gets lessoned. Other organs are used wrongly and eventually become shortened or lengthened. This leads to pain and weakness in many regions of the human anatomy. Your human anatomy farther adjusts or compensates by changing our posture to accommodate to the fluctuations in joints and muscles. Additionally, the limitation in joint movement places additional pressure on the ligaments, muscles and fibrocartilage leading to degenerative joint modifications. The associated joint limitation additionally leads to changed messages being sent and received throughout the nervous system, leading to further aberrations of function and movement. The consequent cycle leads to complex aging of localized muscle and joint tissues. The consequent cycle frequently suppresses easy motion and movement. Statistically, the inability to perform is connected to earlier mortality.

Besides adjustments of movement, our stance, how we balance your human body will be also interrupted. Altered neurological signs from joint dysfunction or restriction allow it to be harder to balance. Research shows that elderly individuals with inadequate balance possess a increased prevalence of drops. What's more, research in the older states that decreasing can be a elevated risk for sooner mortality. Additionally, forward head posture contributes to higher chance of drops. Rounding of their shoulders and also tightening of their anterior torso muscles lead to diminished capacity to breath and could donate to cardio pulmonary issues.

Now it's simple to learn how poor posture, motion and balance might bring about complex aging and sooner departure, however do posture and chiropractic exercise effect that this procedure. Chiropractic works by finding and repairing joints which can be mis aligned and secured. Adjustments restore normal posture and motion inside the combined rendering it less difficult to go. Additionally, the alteration leads to the routine transmission of neural signals from the brain into your human body as well as human body. This ordinary nerve wracking is vital for appropriate balance and muscular contraction, in addition to for the organs to operate correctly. Restoring suitable position into the combined with all the alteration allows for superior alignment of body cells. Chiropractic frequently incorporates acupuncture techniques into regions of muscles leading to the breaking up of adhesions and enhanced motion and endurance. Once the joints have been unlocked and emptied in the alterations, and also the muscles relaxed and stretched by the massage methods, your own body is prepared to be re trained to proceed and hold it self. The effective use of particular postural rehab exercises helps retrain muscles to maneuver correctly and balance exercises help individuals hold our own body at an even far more aligned posture. The mixture of chiropractic adjustments, stretching and massage processes and also exercises that are concentrated permit favorable changes within our balance, movement and recovery. These positive impacts permit us to proceed better even as we age and better accommodate to the outside pressures your system confronts a daily basis. In conclusion, the favorable affects inside the own body as a consequence of the use of posture and chiropractic exercises create a change of these conditions described previously that contribute to premature mortality and aging. As a result of the, posture and chiropractic exercises may be referred to as an anti-fungal therapy.

CHAPTER FOUR

⌘

Natural remedies sciatica

Sciatica is an enormous problem on earth these days. Even though there are lots of diverse treatments for a natural cure for sciatica pain appears to become the ideal. Lots of people seek out an all purely natural remedy but few actually gain in the so called all-natural cure for pain. It's crucial that you learn that sciatica itself just isn't actually a disease, but a disorder triggered by a pair of different illnesses such as a bulging or herniated disk, spinal stenosis, spondylolisthesis, injury, piriformis syndrome, and spinal nerves.

Natural remedy for sciatica

Here we've got some all-natural treatments which could help relieve you of your sciatica pain when properly used along with daily physical exercise.

*juices from berries and celery leaves will provide relief if drunk at minimum number of 10 oz daily. If you put in beet roots and carrots for the mix it is going to get an improved taste and it may also intensify the consequence with the natural remedy.

Decision elderberry tea is really a called muscle relaxant and stimulant and may cure sciatica indications.

*you may also choose garlic nutritional supplements to assist with the pain. In the event you decide to simply take garlic supplements i would advise that you never require a lot more than is reportedly studied on the tag. Consuming raw garlic or taking garlic supplements together with other supplements of vitamin b 1 and complex gives relief from pains and aches, helps flow, is definitely an anti-oxidant and provides your body with warmth and also energy. A great treatment for sciatica is garlic . Only grab two tsp of garlic and then sit in a cup of milk and then beverage this two per day and you'll see results so on.

*another bewitching home remedy to deal with sciatica is brand new minced horseradish poultice, that when put on the painful places and retained for an hour or so at one period arouses the thoracic nerve and also provides immense relief from stomach pain.

A natural treatment for sciatica pain might be quite beneficial but remember to include things like a fantastic eating plan, regular training and also you have to remember that you're intending to boost your general wellbeing. If you would like to avoid with this issue occur again later on you might choose to sleep on a firm mattress. Consistently sit stand in good position, and also stay away from lifting heavy items just as far as feasible. It's the smaller things which cause sciatica pain at the very long haul, therefore make sure you make this part of one's daily routine. Many could find it challenging to stick to those organic patterns.

Sciatica is amongst the common ailments affecting lots of people throughout their life. As stated by the national institutes of health at the USA, it's the 2nd most frequent neurological disorder reported. Only annoyance surpasses it at frequency of reported cases. Its origin is more varied; it may be as naive as a very simple muscle injury or trauma to complicated problems like disk problems, spinal stenosis, osteoporosis, or even cancerous tumors. Oftentimes acupuncture to get sciatica pain alleviation and other organic remedies are all that's required to relieve the pain with the frequent condition.

In case you have spine pain it's sensible to pay for a trip to a own family physician because only your physician can exclude the serious reasons for your back pain. In addition, when addressed and fulfilled head, there's not any sort of sciatica that may not be readily attacked therefore you can find rest from pain.

If, as is likely your pain is the result of a strain or trauma to a lower spine, treatments available are both straightforward and numerous. You also might opt to approach your anxiety in a conventional way, together with exercises to strengthen your heart muscles and treatment drugs or, as the majority are currently doing, process your therapy at a more holistic manner, natural method. On the list of holistic methods accessible are acupuncture, acupuncture, herbal medicine, and noninvasive all-natural methods.

The range of natural remedies, particularly such as trauma or anxiety, offer powerful treatment together with not one of the unwanted shared with medication therapy. Natural methods for treatment tend to be more affordable and more conservative compared to conventional medical procedures to this issue of spine pain. Accepting maids for pain within long spans, as an instance, a conventional strategy, may render you with liver disease, bleeding sores and might even result in death from complications of those unwanted side effects. Some medications relieve pain from dulling pain receptors within your mind. A client of mine that had been on Ultram for pain once clarified the pills because "dumb pills" due to how that it made him feel.

Natural treatments for spine pain

Acupuncture: traditional Chinese medicine including acupuncture because a simple treatment option is dependent on the thought that the chi or life force may get obstructed, which the stations which disperse chi during the human body is able to be discharged through the appropriate insertion of thin needles at the complete points which restrain the chi for the individual complaint. Oftentimes, acupuncture together with a simple program of practice is sufficient to bring back one to pain free residing in a couple weeks.

Eazol: lots of folks swear with this particular natural, cosmetic item. Made of botanical ingredients such as willow bark, lobelia and Boswellia, eazol behaves to lubricate your muscles and also relieve stress in muscular. Additionally, it functions like a safe method to relieve pain.

Yoga: the Indian app of posture meditation and control is a type of exercise which, when directed by a specialist may help relieve the pain of back pain. That isn't any age or sex restriction on the tradition of yoga.

Sexy baths: though ice is ideal for reducing redness, warmth functions to flake out bloated muscle tissues and also behave as a direct supply of relief for the pain. Insert movement like this of a whirlpool and put in sexy tub oils like peppermint or lavender and also the pain-relieving nature of the petroleum adds to this experience. Lots of men and women who take to this adventure hours of aid. Included with some routine of exercise, hot tubs are a really real supply of relief.

Antioxidants and minerals: there are a number of vitamins which are regarded as quite effective for back treatment including vitamin b 12, vitamin, vitamin d, vitamin chamomile along with also others.

Thus there you own it. Natural methods to treatment are a true choice. Acupuncture for sciatica treatment is a high selection but other organic choices may also be offered. Because every situation is different you will need to find which ones work with you. Obviously, remember to always bring exercise for the heart.

People frequently refer shortness pain for a type of disorder, yet this idea is definitely false as this annoyance refers to an undeniable simple fact which you're likely experiencing the herniated disk and also the pain is its own only symptom. Therefore what's the natural treatment for sciatica pain which might be imbibed on your own life to realize some type of relief? Stretches are usually recommended in addition to the ingestion of drugs, but some times is preferred, to assess with a physician or physiotherapist to become certain the exercises have been done precisely.

Celery leaves juices or juices containing potatoes can relieve the pain whenever they're consumed at the number often oz on a normal basis. For those that are already swallowing anti-coagulation drugs or suffering from illnesses like nausea, should choose prior advice from their physician before swallowing the garlic established supplements. If those juices don't agree with your taste buds, and then it is possible to alter your attention to carrot established tea, since it's well known to possess similar sort of ramifications.

Routine ingestion of garlic supplements can't just offer you plenty of energy but in addition, it serves as a superb type of pure cure for pain. Rather than popping vitamin b1 supplements, you also may add foodstuffs such as bread, poultry, legumes, green beans on what you eat in order it helps boost up the degree of vitamin b1 from your system which then can lessen the degree of the sciatica pain.

Sexy and cold packs may perhaps work as wonders because an all-natural cure for pain. Throughout the very first stages of their annoyance, cold packs might also be placed on the affected area for a period of time of roughly twenty-five minutes, often times daily. After a period of a couple of days, you may initiate the using packs and then onwards may utilize both the kinds of packs rather to relieve pain. These packs may enhance the degree of blood flow within your system and consequently it's a successful tool to lower the high level of the stomach pain. With the amalgamation of those herbal treatments it is easy to deal up with the back pain.

Hip anxiety can be quite debatable as it could confine the movement of their human anatomy, treatments may offer relief and also promote smooth and hassle free moves. There are lots of causes of hip pain, so the thigh-bone called femur swivels from the socket in cool to combine top and lower chest of your system and offer joint movement. There's some free space from the socket that gets full of fluid and blood if there's any swelling or disease at the joint. Other structures connected with the joint may be the foundation of annoyance. In the majority of the cases injury is the principal reason for pain. Though stylish pain might be debatable but sometimes referral pain can be also experienced in trendy such as the main one in the instance of irritated thoracic nerve. Arthritis also can trigger hip pain, muscular strain or strained joints can also be commonly found grounds of hip painkillers.

Perhaps not straining the aching section of this trendy throughout the flow while sitting, getting out of bed or bending is just a preventative step to prevent annoyance of this pain. The pain may possibly have been caused because of strained muscle or tendon that may become additional girth if pressure has been exerted onto it throughout any given activity. It may appear that cold and hot compresses would be unable to help as pain is deep inside however it isn't correct, cold and hot compresses could be exceedingly good all-natural cure for hip pain although compressions will likely be implemented for longer duration compared to pain at different regions of the human body. Soft massage in the painful area can be also helpful, pain relieving lotions or gels are also useful for massagetherapy. The massage will likely be achieved with adequate pressure too much nor too much. Massage boosts the flow of blood and therapies swelling and alleviates strained muscles to relieve the pain.

Care may be obtained while sitting and waking out of bed so that an excessive amount of pressure isn't handed down into the bothering location. While sitting softly folding and unfolding straight leg helps if pain is a result of slight overtraining. Leisurely walk wearing horizontal soul shoes is likewise beneficial in boosting the flow of blood and treating discomforts from the fashionable.

Capsaicin ointment can be obtained as over the counter

medicine on the current market and can be an exceptional all-natural pain-relieving lotion. This lotion is composed of pepper that decelerates the signs of pain becoming moved to brain. Ergo a individual feels diminished pain and no pain as a result of its own application. Though this isn't a remedy but respite from pain may aid for making movement and enhancing relaxation.

In case a individual feels shooting pain that's radiating down to thighs compared to this lotion could be helpful because a result a nuisance may result from aggravation of thoracic nerve. Adding the entire body below midsection in bathtub full of heated water and 2 cups of Epsom salt can be a powerful all-natural remedy to relieve hip pain when caused because of muscle cramps or strains. Epsom salt includes calcium that's when consumed by the human body via skin alleviates this type of annoyance. Eating fruits and vegetable, greater ingestion of garlic from your diet, with ginger in foods like in salad along with avoiding red meat and hot food additionally works nearly as good cure for hip pain.

In case you're handling sciatica then you almost certainly understand the pain that's related to that. Handling pain on your back, legs and sometimes even your buttocks could make it rather tricky to work in life. Doing the tiniest tasks might be exceedingly complicated and debilitating. For this reason, you might choose to come across some remedies for sciatica which will work and allow you to relieve the pain.

Naturally, there will be several medications which might succeed when it has to do with decreasing the pain which you will well be experiencing. Some healthcare experts will prescribe anti-inflammatory drugs. The others might enhance muscle relaxants. A lot of people have even found rest out of over-the-counter drugs. You may always should talk with your physician in order they will have the ability to ascertain what kind of medication is going to soon be the right for you personally.

Once the pain has begun to diminish, and you're finding some relief, so you might well be invited to go to physical therapy. You may obtain this to be somewhat useful as the therapist will be in a position to provide you a few programs and exercises which could possibly find a way to help reduce the chance of harms later on. Participants are also educated on what best to improve position and maximize their flexibility in order they don't become injured.

In very acute scenarios, once you aren't getting relief from every other sorts of treatments, your physician might recommend surgery. This program will frequently simply be indicated if you're experiencing fatigue, your intestines are affected with the strain on the guts or your own pain is ongoing to make worse.

Of course, there will be several remedies which you can employ in your home to attempt to diminish the pain which you're having. It might be an advantage to one personally to put a cold pack on the debilitating for about 20 minutes every day. Next, you might find relief should you attempt to substitute cold and heat packs every afternoon. Just ensure you are using your heating pack on the bottom setting.

People who are searching for alternative therapy techniques might decide to try chiropractic services or perhaps acupuncture. It's important to not forget that not all individuals will discover respite from these types of options. Consequently, it's going to be crucial that you take to unique things to find out what's going to help you . You can even talk with your physician prior to hand to see what they can urge.

Natural anti-inflammatories

Pain, swelling, stiffness.. All these are simply a couple words that people use when describing their osteoarthritis. Medicines such as ibuprofen and aspirin can provide quick relief, however they could also result in unwanted side effects when used within a protracted time period. Many vitamin supplements and herbs, by comparison, can provide long-term safe treatment of these pains and pains associated with osteoarthritis. When thinking of a specific nutritional supplement or herb, tips are centered on how much research can be found to encourage its own effectiveness.

Many research studies indicate that glucosamine sulfate supplements can be useful in relieving the symptoms of arthritis. They do so by increasing a jelly-like compound called mucopolysaccharides to boost the shock-absorbing land of joints and inhibiting the elastase receptor, that results in the damage of joints. Studies have also suggested that supplements containing chondroitin sulfate could be helpful; those work by arousing lactic acid, which subsequently increases viscosity from the combined space. If agent turns out to become effective, still another viable choice could be that the nutritional supplement same (s-adenyl methionine). Like glucosamine, sam e is a compound that prevents corrosion of the joint.

Certain herbs may be helpful in the cure of gout. The anti-inflammatory element of devil's claw might offer relief, along with a infusion of avocado/soybean oils was demonstrated to decrease stiffness and pain related to arthritis. Phytodolor is a anti-inflammatory herb mixture made up of ash, aspen and golden rod that could reduce symptoms also. Studies have also demonstrated that niacinamide, a sort of b vitamin based from niacin, might work in relieving pain and swelling. To get a simple and reasonably priced alternative, consider drinking a cup of sour cherry juice each day. Tart cherries are demonstrated to have an potent anti-inflammatory effect, that may be specially valuable in relieving mild cases of arthritis.

Before you go into the retail store, be sure to did your research regarding the services and products that you may be thinking about purchasing. There are tools available offering evaluations and information regarding various herbs and supplements. Bear in your mind to start looking for supplements and never this is the most economical choice; perhaps not all supplements are created equally, and also the most economical supplements aren't always the ideal alternative.

Also remember that seeking the proper treatment solution is dependent upon a individual's individual preferences, demands, along with also condition. Therefore, it is very critical that you consult to your physician before choosing a nutritional supplement or supplement. To initiate the dialog you might state,"i'm interested in choosing supplements. What would you imagine?" this promotes an open conversation and promotes a more collaborative experience along with your medical care provider as a way to ascertain the most effective policy for you.

In present day medicine you will find numerous diverse things which can be utilised to help with treatment for men and women that have chronic reoccurring issues, including lots of all-natural supplements. Certainly one of the most recent improvements to the lineup, maxgxl, supports your entire body's production of glutathione, a enormous anti-inflammatory agent which may definitely offer you a great deal of assistance people who find they're afflicted by issues like rheumatoid arthritis and allergies, which may result in problems when coping with swelling and swelling. This effective anti-oxidant can offer treatment for individuals that have been required to take care of chronic problems for many, many years.

The simple fact that glutathione can be really a enormous anti-inflammatory is another incentive for the many terrific properties. Initially, little was understood about it pure chemical aside from the simple fact it worked wonders being a antioxidant which helped cleanse your body of toxins which was deposited into our systems on a normal basis. But various studies have proven it is often associated with many different crucial roles in the system, pain alleviation being merely one of them. Additionally, it has been discovered that low amounts of atherosclerosis can lead to a individual to degenerate quicker, as their bodies are unable to neutralize the components which accelerate up era factors such as toxins and free radicals.

Because it's been unearthed that treatment can be inserted into this listing of glutathione advantages also, that really is really something of a blessing into the organic medicine armory, especially considering, too, which glutathione is really a enormous anti-aging agent. Once we get older, the creation of pure glutathione in your system reduces therefore to be able to be certain all organs and organs are working in their greatest degrees, it is crucial that you take antidepressant supplements. In reality, lots of have already chose to bring this supplement to their own everyday vitamin regimen to be certain they receive the potent outcomes with the amino acid chemical. Maxgxl is this kind of supplement which supports collagen manufacturing.. And it's natural and organic.

There are certainly a couple common deficiencies which could cause tenderness and sciatica-like pain. A scarcity of all the b vitamins could possibly activate various nerve-related symptoms such as shortness. Of each the b vitamins, lack might be most common in b 6 and b 12. With respect to vitamin b 6 lack, the lack can be due to a lowered ability of your system to convert the vitamin into the active form called pyridoxal-5-phosphate (also called p5p), instead of a deficiency of ingestion of b6. Because of this i suggest having a supplement which comprises at least portion of this b6 from the pyridoxal-5-phosphate sort. From a dose perspective, i would suggest supplementing using 30 to 50 milligrams of pyridoxal-5-phosphate every day. Much like vitamin b 6 lack, vitamin b12 lack is frequently brought more to factors aside from daily ingestion. Vitamin b 12 asks a chemical created by the human body referred to as "intrinsic factor" to be consumed and utilized. Production of inherent variable will frequently be decreased in elderly individuals and those who have a history of alcohol misuse. Because diminished inherent variable prevents the absorption of vitamin b- 12, although supplementation using high oral doses of b 12 in solid shape might well not be enough to fix the lack of in these scenarios, scarcity can be adjusted with periodic shots of liquid vitamin b 12 by a certified health provider, or sub-lingual supplementation. Sub lingual liquid vitamin b12 isn't as easily obtainable as powerful supplements and isn't designed to be consumed, but stored from the mouth under the tongue to get absorption straight into the blood flow during the mucous membranes of your mouth area. Before proceeding using b-12 injections or sub-lingual supplementation, then it's strongly advised that the blood testing has been done in order to ascertain whether there is really a vitamin b12 deficiency. Dosing is dependent upon the concentration of this nutritional supplement used along with the area of the lack of yet another frequent lack that could create sciatica-like outward symptoms is nutrient lack. Fat deficiency is most frequently found in those who lose plenty of fluid during sweat, nausea, vomiting, or nausea, as well as in people with kidney disorder. Additionally, it may occur as a side effect of certain medications, like those for hypertension - notably diuretics. Mild potassium deficiency can typically be adjusted safely simply by gaining more potassium from diet. Even though peanuts would be the traditional high-potassium food, a number of different foods really are of the same quality or even better sources of potassium. These generally include melons, oranges, avocados, many green leafy veggies, and black-strap molasses. Vitamin supplements will also be available, however before taking high doses of vitamins nutritional supplements, it's strongly suggested that blood testing has been performed to quantify cholesterol levels - an excessive amount of potassium may be dangerous! 1 other lack that could make sciatica-like outward symptoms, but usually as part of all-over human body pain, would be co-enzyme q 10 (or even coq-10 for short). This lack is frequently the consequence of a disadvantage of esophageal drugs. There are just two options in tackling the lack. The foremost will be to supplement with coenzyme q 10 at an recommended starting dose of 200 milligrams every day. If it relieves symptoms, then the dose can normally be reduced to 50 to 100 milligrams every day for maintenance. When there isn't any benefit, and symptoms usually do appear to be associated with cholesterol lowering drugs, it's advisable that this issue be discussed with your doctor as well as maybe you are able to switch to an alternative medication or talk alternatives to permit one to log off of this drug altogether. Even though co-enzyme q 10 is generally secure and well-tolerated, it can have the capacity to narrow the bloodstream, and thus if you're on aspirin therapy or even more powerful anabolic medication (for example, coumadin), then you should speak to your health care provider or pharmacist prior to starting pancreatic q 10. In the end, even though perhaps not technically a lack, some diabetics may experience symptoms from the legs which may be confused for sciatica which can be linked to nerve damage resulting from diminished flow. These indicators will often be helped by supplementation with alpha lipoic acid, and it is just a strong anti-inflammatory. For long-term usage, a regular dose of roughly 50 milligrams each day is suggested. Bigger doses are occasionally suggested for short-term usage, but should just be performed under the oversight of a healthcare professional.

Prevention of sciatica

Should you have a pain which awakens out of down your back to a buttock and leg, and then you probably have sciatica. This excruciating pain is due from the most rapid guts of your system termed the sciatic nerve which runs from the back into a buttock and cool and down back of the thighs. It's generally a symptom of some other disease and the length of time it can take for that pain to disappear completely is based upon the reason.

Which exactly are the signs of sciatica? Here are the typical symptoms of the illness:

- you suffer from pain which could differ from a mild annoyance to exceptionally embarrassing. It radiates from the back into a buttock and down the back of the calf and thigh.
- your muscles feel helpless and there can be tingling.
- you get a tingling sensation plus even a pin-and-needles sensation, frequently from the feet.
- symptoms have been aggravated because of prolonged sitting and coughing or coughing.
- there may possibly become described as a lack of bowel or bladder control which requires emergency maintenance.

Which exactly are the causes?

As mentioned previously, this illness requires the sciatic nerve which controls lots of muscles of the calves. If something compresses the origin cause of the nerve located inside the lower back, you go through the signs of sciatica. A herniated disk in the lower spine may be the most frequent reason behind the compression. Disks are made of cartilage and also are observed between the vertebrae in your spine. They act as shock absorbers whenever you proceed. With age, these discs start to deteriorate resulting from the jellylike substance during this disc to float from their outer covering of this disc drive. That is known as disc or herniation. Whilst the herniated disc presses on a nerve root, this causes pain in your leg or back.

Lumbar spinal stenosis, spondylolisthesis, piriformis

syndrome, and adrenal glands are a few of the different illnesses which might result in sciatica.

Age, excessive bending of the spine, taking heavy loads, forcing for lengthy periods, prolonged sitting, and diabetes are a few of the things which put you at a risk with this particular illness.

What's sciatica diagnosed?

Together with rest and time, the illness usually gets improved. But when the pain persists for over one month or becoming progressively more demanding, medical assistance is necessary. Your doctor will conduct an entire physical exam, specially of one's spine and thighs. Some primary tests like walking in your feet or heels will probably be utilised to look at on your muscular strength and girth.

The doctor can suggest an imaging test like a spinal xray, mri, or ct scan when the pain is more intense to eliminate other causes.

The best way to treat sciatica?

Self-care measures like cold or hot packs, overthecounter medications, and extending work well in relieving the symptoms of sciatica. For those who have a herniated disc, then your personal doctor might recommend physical therapy accompanied by rehabilitation therapy once the pain improves. Laughter treatment will contain exercises to strengthen your muscles, and improve your endurance, and adjust your own posture. It's going to assist in preventing recurrent accidents. Prescribed medications like anti-inflammatory medications and muscle relaxants for reducing the redness and relieving the irritation might also be guided by your personal doctor.

Steroidal injections or surgeries like microdiscectomy could possibly be indicated if conservative measures don't alleviate the annoyance.

There are those who've profited by using other remedies like acupuncture, massage, chiropractic, and acupuncture too.

Sciatica therapy exercises can't just maintain your spine healthy later on, but might work to get back pain at this time in the event that you realize the proper ones and also how to complete them. In the event you suffer with sciatica, then you're no stranger to this pain this illness might cause. Maybe you simply take control the counter or prescription pain relievers, however you have to be aware there is yet another, more natural means to alleviate the pain and also protect against upcoming sciatica pain permanently. Many caregivers advise that you start exercising instantly, since this really is the very best approach to find the treatment you require. Thus, escape bed and start curing your spine and relieving your back pain.

Sciatica anxiety is due when the nerves have been rubbed or compacted. This may lead to an unpleasant burning sensation that runs down the leg into the foot and frequently the pain may become so acute it could be hard to go. This is exactly the reason why nausea exercises are therefore essential, because they function to fortify either side of the spine muscles and also prevent pulling of their spine in any one direction. This assist keep the spine correctly coordinated and protect against prospective stress on the sciatic nerve.

Not just in the event you're doing sciatica training

exercises to avoid your pain today, however it is necessary to adopt an everyday workout routine that targets keeping the heart and spine muscles strong and that means it's possible to prevent future troubles with your digestive tract wracking. In the event you are afflicted with disk troubles, then you will likely even discover that a fantastic solid exercise routine could continue to keep them healthy as well and this may prevent problems like slipped and herniated discs.

Just what exactly sciatica therapy exercises if you be doing today?

Exercises which will fortify your'heart' with muscle relaxation therapy, however, can train your muscles to take part as a way to assist one to remain healthy and powerful. They're a terrific method to be certain the spine and heart are both robust and equipped to interact to maintain your body moving without injury to either disks or the plantar nerve.

Now you also need to think of sciatica exercises which enable one to extend your spine muscles. Since the spine muscles may grow at different speeds and one negative can be stronger, it generates tenseness from the trunk. As time passes, these stressed muscles will tug in the backbone and may create stress on the stomach muscles. By doing sciatica exercises, then you also are able to keep your muscles prevent yanking both sides, and this could continue to keep your spine straight and impartial.

When done each day, such as contraceptive treatment exercises can enable one to own a powerful, pain-free back and core to lifetime, regardless of what you end up doing.

CHAPTER FIVE

✑

The solution to prevention and recovery

With the exclusion of these few cases whenever there is structural damage to the true spine due to bulging disks or spinal stenosis, exercises for sciatica treatment would be just the ticket that you require for a comprehensive recovery. In the rare instances of structural triggers of the low backpain, strengthening the heart muscles might assist you to avert or, at the lowest, delay more revolutionary operation.

The center muscle tissue which encourage that the backbone are usually one of the most neglected muscle groups from your system yet these muscles, even should cared of regularly, offer you the best prevention against toenails readily available. What's more astonishing is the fact that the exercises demanded can be achieved before you get out of bed each daytime. Ten minutes each day and you also decrease the danger of back pain significantly.

Next-to chronic headache, back pain and tenderness pain has become really the most familiar of most neurological disorders based on the national institutes of health. As it's very prevalent, lots of men and women wonder why there's not any fantastic means to safeguard against the distress and pain due to inflammation of the sciatic nerve. Well, there's and it surely works. Becoming proactive by strengthening your heart muscles in addition to extending encourage muscle tissues, putting them into very good condition, helps encourage the majority of one's own weight and eliminates stress or injury related back pain.

Look, i am not talking about developing six-pack muscles . What i am speaking about is clearly basic conditioning; strengthening and conditioning the ab muscles, the obliques, hip adductors and abductors and hip flexors at the exact minimum combined side stretching hamstrings and in addition the muscles at the base is all that's required to reduce overtraining or, even if it occurs, to accelerate recovery at the fantastic bulk of cases. The purpose is it is the center which enables one to drift up on two-legs, to flex in addition to twist, so to sit readily, to lift to complete those activities which make you human. Caring for the critical muscle band has to be a top priority.

In case your goal would be to protect against the occurrence of menstruation afterward employed by 2-3 weeks using a fitness expert on developing a easy routine for your center is a fantastic idea. The workouts to the back and heart can be specific and also there are a great deal of muscles included. Attempting to generate a schedule by yourself can do more damage while in the future compared to just good. For certain, in the event that you presently have back pain then speak with your doctor and receive a referral to a physical therapist who will help you through the very ideal workout routine for relieving your discomfort. In a nutshell, do not make an effort to take care of your spine by yourself. Search expert guidance as it really is that essential.

No matter if you're performing exercises to state that the heart so as to relieve chronic back pain, then it's necessary to get them on the normal basis. If your objective is clearly pain relief, then you ought to achieve your exercises even in the event that you're damaging. Why is it conducive is your data that conditioning and strengthening the true core reduces your recovery period somewhat? The additional bonus of quitting a recurrence of this sciatica is really a long-term incentive based in the own effort. When performing exercises for sciatica start off at a traditional manner. There's not any requirement to test to do everything simultaneously. Since your heart gets more sturdy add many walking, mowing the lawn, cardio and swimming in case you have a mind to achieve that. A powerful core supplies you with options which you cannot create whenever your heart has gone outside of illness.

All these days many caregivers recommend exercises for sciatica. Actually, the absolute best caregivers will supply you with a special, customized exercise program built round the root reason behind one's own sciatica. The goal of the exercise is twofold. Firstly, to relieve the instantaneous short term sciatic pain and second to construct your strength and state to protect against some future flare-ups of sciatica.

Even though most peoples first urge is to simply take with their own bed when struck sciatica, anything outside a few days mattress rest really does more damage than good. The shortage of movement is awful to the joints and the bones which donate to your own esophagus and will result in distress and lack of conditioning, and which subsequently may cause future traumas and much more annoyance.

When i said earlier in the day, ideally your work out regime will be tailored especially to your inherent problem that resulted in the sciatica. However, almost any app for prevention and relief of sciatica could incorporate these elements.

Stretches: stretching of these essential muscles within the field is very important; this can even boost the freedom of the joints and ligaments. You need to focus on this hamstring, the muscles behind your thighs, and also the piriformis muscle, which then runs throughout the buttocks. The stretches in many cases are removed from yoga and consuming full dismissed yoga is an advantage to all thoracic victims.

Core strengthening: the heart muscles of the spine and gut have to be strong as you possibly can in whoever has suffered any kind of spine problem. When there's a fault with the backbone, powerful heart muscles may help encourage that weakness. Once more yoga exercises are all good, but many physiotherapists urge pilates and also a lot of core-strengthening can be accomplished using a gym ball, fit ball or even swiss-ball. Which can be the exact same task, however, understood by an assortment of titles.

Aerobic exercise: this may aid with overall fitness, endurance and strength. However, you are going to wish to avert any superior impact exercise which can nourish the spine and cause you further problems. Swimming and walking would be ideal. The generally accepted target for walking will be usually to be in a position to reach 3 kilometers (5 kms) each day in a lively pace. But make sure you gradually develop for the when it's not used for you.

Form: " it nearly goes without saying, but you should be confident you are doing exactly the exercises properly, in proper shape. If you can cause further issues on the spine and sciatic nerve-wracking. If you've got somebody instruction you originally and viewing your own form. If that isn't possible, make certain that you follow some directions and diagrams into the correspondence.

Effective sciatica nerve treatment

I personally might love to supply you with the signs of sciatica. In this way you're going to have the ability to be aware of in case you've got it. Afterward, i will follow what the majority of individuals do to treatments. Finally, i will provide you an extra treatment others do - that's come to be the best and safe treatment for carry.

Sciatica occurs whenever there's aggravation to the thoracic nerve whenever there's degeneration of the low thoracic disks. When the disks are all worn, then the bone of the vertebra pinches the guts. Once the vertebrae is out of alignment that the manhood at which the guts is gets pinched.

From the gluteus maximus (buttocks) there's a muscle known as the piriformis. The thoracic should put under your muscle. But, there are instances when it really is finished the piriformis, also, on infrequent occasions, cut through the muscle.

Throughout improper diet that's mostly acidic rather than alkaline, there's a shortage of calcium at the disks. The disks also get there or stretchable might be described as a prolapsed disk.

In this degenerated say the border of these vertebrae just isn't eloquent and flat however, "teeth-like". Together with your spine out of alignment, there's a pull the piriformis. While this occurs, the piriformis muscle can pinch and then irritate nerve.

The pain could begin from the buttocks or it might stretch the leg down entirely into the heels. If you're experiencing this sort of pain, then you probably have time consuming.

A number of the feeling you might happen are: tingling, burning, tingling sensation at the leg and thigh. The condition can be so debilitating it gets it tough to walk

Most people picked a debilitating surgery in their own vertebrae but in accordance with dr. James Weinstein, a professor of orthopedic surgery in Dartmouth university, maintained a surgery isn't powerful. His analysis had been based on 2000 patients who'd ruptured disks and contrasted to people have been medicated non-surgically.

Some people today assert that self-improvement works in families, it doesn't. Why is it seem that it works in families could be the exact identical way of life? When eating customs are identical, and that they truly are for huge numbers of men and women, it contributes to the "same cause and effect."

There are approximately 300,000 Americans who experience a surgery in their own vertebrae. Thus, in consequence, in line with dr. Weinstein, they're better than people that cope with sciatica in different ways.

Who will be most probably influenced?

People between the ages of 25-45 really have a issue using their vertebrae. Early correction of their vertebrae and appointment on life styles would be your better prevention for sciatica.

The sciatic nerve could be the largest from the body therefore that it mustn't looked within treatment. The aggravation is normally happened as a consequence of the misalignment of the vertebrae. Someone could get their bottoms out of alignment, not comprehend it suffer some pain - at early phases. For that reason, individuals have a tendency to dismiss a checkup.

A side from operation, a frequent kind of treatment is drugs, specifically, pain killers. Painkillers are awful on the kidneys and also, needless to say, it will not arrive at the explanation for the pain.

Some alternative treatments

To get better choices to this treatment of sciatic you can find lots of alternatives.

Eat a foods full of garlic, garlic, ginger and kelp. These herbs are referred to as anti-inflammatory.

Drink 68 glasses of plain water that's been filtered. This will avoid muscle cramps. You can't rely on coffee, tea and beverages as plain water whenever you're calculating your 6 8 drinks. This will look after the stiffness and stiffness related to sciatica.

Exercise is yet still another fantastic option. Specifically, a fitness in which you increase up your knees to your chest area. Good stretching of these thighs is effective, too.

Finally, lots of men and women that have sciatica will go to a professional of quantum-touch. Some physicians and osteopaths are currently incorporating this therapy inside their own practice. This treatment only entails a mild touch of their palms within the affected region and total treatment is preferred with most customers later one session.

Benefits of exercise for people with sciatica

Acute sciatic nerve pain may appear to be ineffective occasionally, therefore that I discovered ways to repair my sciatica. To get started using for a long time i would like to work with a heating system to use to relieve the pain however, once i removed heat the pain was there as awful or a few times worse. I then learned this, to repair my burnout, " i have to happen to be using icepacks for twenty five minutes every a couple of hours (this helped manner more compared to warmth) and followed with exercises intended to extend back and forth the pain which has been running down my thighs into the back, that really help hasten the healing procedure.

Should you be afflicted by acute back pain which runs down your buttocks, thighs and all of the way to your feet, then odds are that you suffer from sciatica. If you really don't understand what this really is, it's pain from the digestive tract being pinched damaged or using pressure placed onto it in many diverse sources.

Once i unearthed my spine pain was a result of a pinched sciatic nerve i began to search for means to repair my sciatica by understanding exactly what the guts was where it had been located within my physique. The sciatic nerve is upper nerve in our bodies, which begins from the spinal cord and also goes throughout the vertebrae and disks of the spinal cord down throughout the buttock down the thighs all of the way to your feet, why your feet sometimes tingle or feel helpless as well when undergo intense sciatica.

Now let us take a look at a few of things which cause sciatic nerve pain and damage:

- improper lifting of heavy items (here really is actually the top reason for this nerve damage)
- rust of the back because of aging
- pinching of the nerve because back injury such like, herniated or smashed disks
- degenerative disk disease
- pressure in the nerve from nerves swelling or swelling as a result of a busted piriformis muscle (this muscular is lean and attaches to the lower back runs down the buttocks and attaches into the thighbone, the sciatic nerve works beneath this muscle) this popularly called piriformis syndrome
- growing tumors in the backbone in the region of the nerve putting strain onto it
- a misaligned back

Knowing what exactly the guts is and where it's located caused it to be simpler for me personally to discover strategies to repair my sciatica, like i mentioned earlier in the day heat was the incorrect means to alleviate the pain, also perhaps not exercising which extended and concentrated the pain left the pain persist more. Once i began itself treatments that i came across within a e book referred to as "sciatica self-maintenance" i discovered that i relieve the pain faster and keep it from recurring in the foreseeable future. On certain occasions i discovered this to repair my toenails demanded a physician to re align the spine to relieve the strain on the guts afterward, with the correct exercises that i really could continue to keep the spine in alignment and block the sciatica from coming.

Yoga exercises

Who's wouldn't normally like to find yoga at no cost? Exactly like every one, you too could be enthusiastic about this way collection of free yoga exercises which are meant only for you! All these yoga practice will teach you on the best way best to exercise yoga; you simply must follow the directions carefully with full confidence.

Ashtanga yoga is really a string of unique kinds of exercises that ought to be practiced regularly to enhance somebody's health. Exercising raises the critical stream of energy and supplies a reassurance. The absolutely free exercises listed here are only different poses that will need to become practiced properly.

Yoga is additionally a method of alive. It features performing daily routine tasks at a normal period regular. Consider the habit of getting up in the daytime. In yoga, the everyday routine starts with the a predetermined procedure of exercise regular in three different points; original, japa significance knocking a few headline over and up to keep up exactly the exact comprehension; secondly, study by reading a few yoga programs; and next, meditation that ought to really be performed in a predetermined period in a predetermined place regular.

The initial present of these absolutely free yoga exercises needs to function as that the corpse pose, and also be replicated between other asana (yoga poses) so that as your last comfort. This present looks easy and it's really quite fine too. However, it ought to be useful for a lot more than just relaxing. You ought to utilize this particular pose for meditation when allowing the mind to obtain relax and strength.

Start those yoga exercises with a warmup exercises to relax and prepare your muscles to the upcoming exercises.

After warm you up can carry out the shoulder lifts the natural after exercise and also a person's attention, and this can enhance your eyesight and protect against fatigue. For the upcoming exercises you may practice sun salutation that'll extend all of your body tissues, this to organize for the far harder exercises. Attempt also leg lift, that'll tone your leg muscles, so providing you with longer endurance and improved flexibility; mind rack posture is also decent for resting several of one's organs like heart.

As soon as you prepare your body and mind for longer challenging yoga practice, begin in the next manner.

Start with the bridge along with plough presents; this can improve your back's endurance. Initially, you might find it tough to reach the last position. However, with exercise you'll have the ability to accomplish this"asana". In the beginning you won't have the capacity to execute it but remember it is vital that you attempt and make it to the ideal location and train your own body to finally reach the absolutely balanced posture.

Later this pose, try out the forward bend present to excite the nervous system. Afterward it's possible to attempt the fish present, it strengthens the torso lungs and muscles.

Next pose is known as cobra pose. Women who have problems with degenerative issues might try out the cobra present, it arouses the pelvic and lower abdominal region, improving the flow and massaging the body organs.

Should you want to reinforce the back, then you definitely need to try out the locust pose. Locust pose is known to help prevent constipation.

The bow is just still another present to assist your spine area stay powerful and flexible at precisely the exact same period along with abdominal fat my additionally be reduced when the proper diet is put on. Furthering this yoga practice you are able to try out the half twist pose for the spines.

Breathing is an extremely essential aspect in practicing yoga. You're able to learn appropriate method of breathing and enhance it by practicing exactly the crow pose. With this particular present, you are able to better your arm and joints stamina too. Afterward it is possible to try out the hands to foot pose and also the triangle. This pose necessitates the strength and flexibility.

At the end of most of these yoga exercise exercises; be certain you do the corpse present to recover any energy that's been lost throughout these totally free yoga practice also to offer rest to the entire body.

You are able to decide to try these completely free yoga exercises by one and watch for yourself that one's work the right for you personally. Knowing the poses which benefit you, only ensure you usually do not over stretch yourself into doing those exercises also that you observe exactly the exact same pair of exercises regularly.

Should you are considering taking a sort of practice with the purpose of creating yourself feel and look far better that you have to give very serious thought to yoga.

Yoga works in your human body and mind and its results is understood in lots of diverse aspects - within our own bodies, their own health insurance and the way they look, and on our heads - how we view the planet.

Therefore just how do yoga exercises change from other kinds of exercise?

Yoga exercises, also called asanas or postures, are put on the full body of the body. Alternatively,

Lots of other workout regimes really are a sort of technology placed on the muscles of their human body. Which usually means that yoga exercises are more worried about more than simply the shallow growth of muscles. The bearings utilized in yoga exercises have a tendency to normalize the purposes of the full organism.

The advantage of yoga exercises is they could modulate the involuntary processes of respiration and help the flow and digestion, elimination and metabolism etc. The exercises also function to impact the working of the glands and glands, in addition to the nervous system and also your head. This outcome is reached by doing heavy breathing as your system is put into a variety of postures. Every one of those yoga exercises creates an alternative totality from the connection that is functional inside the organism.

Thus, yoga can influence person physically, emotionally, morally and emotionally. Yoga highlights the doctrine of exercise. Under its training experiences a feeling of awakening. Each one's abilities are more heightened, and yet one accomplishes equilibrium and endurance through these aerobic exercises, some of which are modeled following the movements of different

Creatures. In aerobic exercises, comfort is educated as a art, breathing for being a science, and emotional control of your human body for a way of harmonizing the body, mind, and soul.

The advanced stages of yoga require several years of special preparation-practices. Now's manner of living, its pace and environment, imply this is tricky to realize. But, practicing yoga, yoga and heavy breathing and relaxation methods, with some of the period dedicated to meditation and concentration is some thing

Everyone could reach.

Yoga exercises may have a beneficial impact on those that suffer from illness or disease. Whilst it isn't ready to cure those matters, practicing yoga may implies that obstacles and impurities have been removed to ensure nature may do its curative work.

Therefore, if you're searching for a sort of exercise is effective favorably on your system and mind, and also something which is relatively simple to squeeze in to a daily routine then not consume exercises. The expanding prevalence of yoga exercises ensures you will likely locate a yoga center or some gymnasium that provides local classes in your town. If, nevertheless, you don't need enough time for you to attend classes you'll find lots of novels and dvd's on aerobic exercises, which means that you may perform it in your home at some period if it's suitable for you personally.

Within just a day or two of performing yoga exercises it's likely to come to feel revitalized as well as more healthy. Continued training of yoga exercises may make us fitter and more joyful.

The ideal in indian conventional kind of exercising is

meditation that can supply a helpful way by that to boost your brain and the soul within and adds essential strength to your individual's human body and it all needs to gain from yoga will be really to master about the appropriate bearings in addition to methods of breathing. Ostensibly, everyone may do yoga practice provided that they have a very yoga mat and also actually, should they ensure selecting the suitable yoga mat, then they also are able to enjoy greater and a lot more comfortable at the exact same time as relaxing cycling practice.

Earlier you choose a particular yoga practice mat tote it pays to you to have a look at the different available yoga exercises mats and also the truth is, choosing a eco-yoga physical exercise mat is likely to soon be wise since the one that's surely built from pvc will place your health in danger and so needs to be avoided because a wonderful bargain as you possibly can.

One in the accessories that are essential to save your mat is truly a yoga mat tote which also helps you take your yoga mat together with you where you move. In reality, the better yoga mats could be folded along with wrapped and those are able to be placed within a yoga mat tote and performed with you too as useful for keeping your yoga exercises mat whilst it isn't being used.

An excellent yoga mat tote should be capable of carrying out a significant yoga mat which can measure up to hundred inches and additionally the yoga mat tote is good fitted to carrying along on your own journeys plus in addition, it helps assure the mat remains comfy and is protected from the weather and naturally, out of dirt.

You are able to find quite a-few diverse styles from which to choose if it concerns a superb yoga mat tote and the one which you opt for will be dependent on the size at precisely the exact same period as fabric employed and depends upon its layouts and you'll discover also various models for you to elect choose pick from. The simple truth is that it's rather typical to run into that yoga practice mat totes are made from silk and sometimes cotton whereas people manufactured out of jute as well as oftentimes velvet may also be rather well-known.

You want to create sure the yoga exercises mat tote that you want on buying is lasting plus it needs to be hardy enough to resist normal damage and in addition, it might likewise encourage to have a very yoga mat tote that's watertight, also for everyone these features, a handbag made from cotton will probably soon be most suitable.

If it concerns a yoga mat handbag constructed from lace or silk, they'll generally have cotton liner (thick) which contributes to their durability too as durability and several have very interesting patterns and comprise vibrant colors too as possess brilliant textures and are appropriate to people that need something out in your standard.

Yoga exercises would be the perfect way to spare your mind also to focus heavily. As soon as you've seen a stressful situation, the thoughts, body and soul is worn outside and exhausted. The reason of them may possibly have been out of the interaction with different people or something which have resulted in a pity, anger, melancholy and disappointment in you personally. These feelings generated out of those circumstances needs to be published so you may live a more joyful life. 1 effective method and also way expressing your own outpoured feelings and feelings is by simply doing yoga exercises. Once you truly feel like crying aloud or breaking the tv, you're able to as an alternative release your anxiety through yoga exercises which can be effective and beneficial. Such a plan has functioned in lots of ways for diverse men and women. People of us who do not find sufficient time for themselves may perform yoga exercises as a way to relieve themselves. Sometimes, work has captured us up so closely we do not find time for you to curl up and state ourselves. Yoga exercises are among the better remedies for this issue. Yoga exercises might also be implemented and heard from school. There are a number of sessions offering yoga clinics. The exercises you'll see in school might be performed in your home. In reality, you are able to learn a few yoga exercises in home by yourself. You are only going to need to desire a tv and a videotape. The tape reveals the following steps and steps for each yoga practice. Throughout a weary and heavy daytime, you also may set just a small commitment and time in doing aerobic exercises. Also bear in mind that in doing yoga, then you will have to be persistent in practicing the exercises in order it will soon take effect and you'll find over time developments in your own entire body. After doing the yoga exercises, then you ought to curl up for the consequence of those positions occur place. This way, your system will collect the outcomes. Before doing the yoga exercises, then you ought to lay at a relaxed posture which means that you may focus well and never be diverted by outside forces. You won't feel discomfort or pain too. Yoga exercises may be done anytime of the time provided that you're free. Even though it selects virtually no moment, still, the very best time to clinic it really is each daytime. Before eating your breakfast, then your mind is dependent upon its condition of calmness and clear of distractions. This really may be the best time to accomplish exercises. Before doing the exercises, make certain the heart is ready. It ought not feel any self or pain. It's crucial to maintain a fantastic center which means your brain can get the job done well. The right spot to accomplish your yoga exercises would be a silent location. It ought to be well ventilated and free of most of disagreeable things as well as smell. You ought to be liberated of all probable distractions. Keeping a fantastic tummy can be crucial therefore you may feel well along with your gastrointestinal tract answers accurately. What you ought to do is to drain your intestines and clean your noses. You ought to stay fit and clean. Now you have obviously understood the critical reminders, then you can begin your yoga exercises and work out your way.

Yoga is among the exercises which have boundless health and fitness benefits; by the robust and elastic body, a calm mind, a luminous beautiful skin, fat reduction for healing. It gives immense benefits which not only joins your system, but additionally boosts your head in addition to the breathing strategy. It compels stability and leaves your life more serene, happier and fulfilling.

Routine yoga training will give you with all around fitness center. This suggests you won't you should be getting physically healthy; however, you'll also be receiving mentally and mentally fit throughout the exercises. That is authorized by different exercises such as positions, breathing methods and meditation which yoga comprises.

Now you can even shed weight with yoga in the event that

you're too heavy or in the event that you only need to drop some weight to better the physique. Once you take out yoga clinics, you'll begin becoming sensitive regarding the foods which you will likely be giving your entire body and the perfect time you'll be carrying foods. While doing so, you'll be keeping tabs on your own weight reduction.

Yoga methods can allow you to relieve stress that collects daily. With only a couple of minutes of yoga, then you will really feel liberated on the own body in addition to mind from some other stress which you may be going right through. The yoga poses, meditation and also the breathing processes can assist you to overcome tension and melancholy. In an advanced level yoga grade, it is possible to even utilize yoga exercises to detoxing your system and de-stressing mind.

Still another health advantage you can receive from yoga exercises will be inner peace. When a few folks desire inner serenity, they see quite places rich in natural magnificence. Nonetheless, it's also great to be aware you could experience inner peace anywhere you might be and in any given moment. As an example, doing yoga exercises on your house will be able to assist you to get the inner peace that's available right in it. You do not necessarily need to attend a particular spot to have it. Inner-peace is quite essential in calming a troubled mind.

Now you may also gain from improved resistance if you execute routine exercises. For the body to get the job done well, your body mind and soul require to blend together. When there was an irregularity within your system, your head is going to be influenced inducing to experience guilt or unpleasantness. The yoga poses can also enable you to strengthen your muscles and also massage your own muscles. Besides relieving you in stress, breathing and meditation techniques may even enhance your own immunity.

Routine Pilates exercises can make the own body to own better posture and flexibility. Should you really miss a human body that's strong, flexible and supple, the trick is to add yoga in your ordinary routine. The own body tissues will be elongated and tone plus they'll become stronger. The own body posture once you stand, sit, sleep or walk will probably be made better. In the event that you will often possess human body aches because of incorrect position, yoga methods may assist you to overcome them.

Now you may likewise feel pumped up with energy in the event you maintain routine exercises. Should you feel tired out by the ending of your afternoon, or you also detect taking out multiple activities to become quite tiring, a couple minutes of exercising every day will make you feeling lively and fresh daily. Throughout your afternoon, you'll likely be refreshed and prepared to execute those activities of daily.

When you execute yoga exercises frequently, and you will establish greater intuition. Meditation can enhance your instinctive capability and permit one to comprehend cheaply what ought to be achieved, how it has to be achieved and exactly what period it has to be carried out. This can allow you to yield very good outcomes or boost your performance in your everyday pursuits.

In early India, yoga has been a method of living that comprised moral, moral, religious, and physiological components. Postures (asana) were also an essential, but tiny sector of the early clinic. Today, a lot of men and women make use of the word "yoga" to mean a certain sort of physical exercise, even while being totally oblivious of its own spiritual part, making the present-day model of meditation a shadow of its former self. Some classes wind without a time spent from the worthiness of pranayama, relaxation, or meditation.

To put it yet another way, the vital yoga mat, utilized in today's exercise variant, could just be needed to get a modest part of a genuine yoga clinic. As stated by maharishi Patanjali's writings, at the yoga sutras, asana is simply among eight limbs over yogic philosophy - most which can be utilized to organize for the greatest marriage of someone's inner intellect together with worldwide comprehension. As stated by proponents of conventional yoga, it's not possible to accomplish enlightenment simply by doing a bodily practice, even when a person practices the very complex postures.

In addition to providing a twisted view of this original clinic, contemporary yoga was sidetracked and used as a procedure to market popularity and sell pictures to people. This consists of personal stardom, and any such thing from correct organic mats, for high priced high style accessories and clothing. While this isn't inherently bad whatsoever, it scarcely looks like the humble way of life, and unwavering dedication, of those numerous sages, who retained yoga living for generations throughout Sanskrit texts and oral teachings. When yogic teachings gained worldwide awareness, it was just natural to modern yoga to simply take its own individuality.

This doesn't follow that the bodily exercises at modern meditation are poor or some less efficient compared to people at different tasks. In reality, asanas and leaks maybe more powerful than a number of different sorts of exercise. Studies have revealed that yoga movement improves physical health and fitness, help prevent illness, reduce depression and stress, reduce anxiety, promote comfort, and an overall awareness of wellbeing. Purists, however, could wonder if these fitness-based styles ought to really be called yoga.

The fact remains that few folks in the 21stcentury, are most likely to devote long intervals at ashrams because apprentices, meditating, and living the life span of some conventional yogi. In reality, a little bit of yoga is definitely greater than no yoga in any way. If modern yoga exercises is really helping create a more healthy and more peaceful society, also reducing the amazing price of health care bills, it's magic in itself.

Still another issue with modern yoga is that the significantly confusing actuality that a few folks think it to be counterproductive with their own religious beliefs or opinion systems. Meditation is a life style, not just a religion. Yoga doesn't discriminate. It will not look to hinder human beliefs or rationale, and anybody is welcome to appreciate its benefits. Afterall, who can assert with a fitter, happier, more peaceful planet?

The exercise is imagined to loosen the central nervous system and also stabilize the whole human body, mind, and soul. It's thought with its own enthusiasts to steer clear of certain ailments. Doing this type of exercise usually help make the human body's immune mechanisms strong assisting your own body to be in a position to manage lots of disorders like annoyance, fatigue and so forth. The curative rate of a personal accident or only a wound can be additionally enhanced. In addition, yoga practice was employed to lessen hyper tension degrees, reduce stress, and boost coordination, endurance, attention, sleeping, and food digestion. Medical professionals along with scientists have been researching latest the huge benefits of exercising regularly. Studies demonstrate that it might potentially decrease the signs of many popular and sometimes life-threatening disorders including arthritis, arteriosclerosis, acute fatigue, diabetes, obesity, aids, asthma attack along with weight loss issues.

Together with treating disorders, yoga practice is presently one among the choices for drugs. Together with yoga exercises like a combination of physical exercises, breathing exercises, and meditation, it turns to a specially effective type of physical activity for people that have certain medical difficulties. For anyone who have cardiovascular disease, various studies have proven yoga practice to aid people young and old. In particular, the exercise appears to enhance cardiovascular disease in lots of ways, including controlling elevated blood pressure rates and increasing immunity to emotional stress. Scientific tests made at yoga establishments in india have recorded impressive success in relieving asthma. Additionally, it has been proven that asthma conditions can normally be prevented by way of yoga courses without turning into medicinal drugs. Yoga can be thought to decrease pain by helping the brain's pain center regulates the gate-controlling system found in the back and also the release of natural pain killers in the physique. Cardiovascular exercises utilized in yoga additionally can reduce strain. Considering the fact that muscles have a tendency to curl up once you breathe, widening time of exhalation can help provide comfort decreasing strain. Recognizing breathing helps to acquire calmer, less fast respiration and help with comfort and pain control. Yoga has got the chance to buffer against the damaging impact of physiological self-objectification also to build up embodiment and wellbeing.

Moreover, the practice was broadly studied as a way in lowering (and occasionally remove) many cardiovascular risks. A number of these unwanted side effects include lower the circulation of blood, renal system failure, menopausal failure, as well as blindness. Many researchers believe practicing yoga and with daily aid services and products on a frequent basis might help stimulate blood circulation and massage tissues, which regularly can offer long-term bodily advantages to people fighting diabetes. In addition, the practice of yoga may provide long-term benefits for those who have diabetes because this was ascertained to decrease sugar levels, obtaining a fantastic result on every kind of diabetes, including type 1 and type 2 diabetes.

Yoga exercise is actually the very best medicine for several sort of health issues and also a very excellent refresher of individual brain, body and soul. It helps to get a person emotionally and emotionally productive. Consequently, everyone should start performing yoga exercise often to remain healthy and fit to very existence.

Acute sciatic nerve pain may appear to be ineffective occasionally, therefore that i discovered ways to repair my sciatica. To get started using for a long time i would like to work with a heating system to use to relieve the pain however, once i removed heat the pain was there as awful or a few times worse. I then learned this, to repair my burnout, " i have to happen to be using icepacks for twenty five minutes every a couple of hours (this helped manner more compared to warmth) and followed with exercises intended to extend back and forth the pain which has been running down my thighs into the back, that really help hasten the healing procedure.

Should you be afflicted by acute back pain which runs down your buttocks, thighs and all of the way to your feet, then odds are that you suffer from sciatica. If you really don't understand what this really is, it's pain from the digestive tract being pinched damaged or using pressure placed onto it in many diverse sources.

Once i unearthed my spine pain was a result of a pinched sciatic nerve i began to search for means to repair my sciatica by understanding exactly what the guts was where it had been located within my physique. The sciatic nerve is upper nerve in our bodies, which begins from the spinal cord and also goes throughout the vertebrae and disks of the spinal cord down throughout the buttock down the thighs all of the way to your feet, why your feet sometimes tingle or feel helpless as well when undergo intense sciatica.

Now let us take a look at a few of things which cause sciatic nerve pain and damage:

- improper lifting of heavy items (here really is actually the top reason for this nerve damage)
- rust of the back because of aging
- pinching of the nerve because back injury such like, herniated or smashed disks
- degenerative disk disease
- pressure in the nerve from nerves swelling or swelling as a result of a busted piriformis muscle (this muscular is lean

and attaches to the lower back runs down the buttocks and attaches into the thighbone, the sciatic nerve works beneath this muscle) this popularly called piriformis syndrome

- growing tumors in the backbone in the region of the nerve putting strain onto it
- a misaligned back

Knowing what exactly the guts is and where it's located caused it to be simpler for me personally to discover strategies to repair my sciatica, like i mentioned earlier in the day heat was the incorrect means to alleviate the pain, also perhaps not exercising which extended and concentrated the pain left the pain persist more. Once I began itself treatments that i came across within a e book referred to as "sciatica self-maintenance" I discovered that i relieve the pain faster and keep it from recurring in the foreseeable future. On certain occasions I discovered this to repair my toenails demanded a physician to re align the spine to relieve the strain on the guts afterward, with the correct exercises that i really could continue to keep the spine in alignment and block the sciatica from coming.

Yoga exercises

Who's wouldn't normally like to find yoga at no cost? Exactly like every one, you too could be enthusiastic about this way collection of free yoga exercises which are meant only for you! All these yoga practice will teach you on the best way best to exercise yoga; you simply must follow the directions carefully with full confidence.

Ashtanga yoga is really a string of unique kinds of exercises that ought to be practiced regularly to enhance somebody's health. Exercising raises the critical stream of energy and supplies a reassurance. The absolutely free exercises listed here are only different poses that will need to become practiced properly.

Yoga is additionally a method of alive. It features performing daily routine tasks at a normal period regular. Consider the habit of getting up in the daytime. In yoga, the everyday routine starts with the a predetermined procedure of exercise regular in three different points; original, japa significance knocking a few headline over and up to keep up exactly the exact comprehension; secondly, study by reading a few yoga programs; and next, meditation that ought to really be performed in a predetermined period in a predetermined place regular.

The initial present of these absolutely free yoga exercises needs to function as that the corpse pose, and also be replicated between other asana (yoga poses) so that as your last comfort. This present looks easy and it's really quite fine too. However, it ought to be useful for a lot more than just relaxing. You ought to utilize this particular pose for meditation when allowing the mind to obtain relax and strength.

Start those yoga exercises with an warmup exercises to relax and prepare your muscles to the upcoming exercises. After warm you up can carry out the shoulder lifts the natural after exercise and also a person's attention, and this can enhance your eyesight and protect against fatigue. For the upcoming exercises you may practice sun salutation that'll extend all of your body tissues, this to organize for the far harder exercises. Attempt also leg lift, that'll tone your leg muscles, so providing you with longer endurance and improved flexibility; mind rack posture is also decent for resting several of one's organs like heart.

As soon as you prepare your body and mind for longer challenging yoga practice, begin in the next manner.

Start with the bridge along with plough presents; this can improve your back's endurance. Initially, you might find it tough to reach the last position. However, with exercise you'll have the ability to accomplish this "asana". In the beginning you won't have the capacity to execute it but remember it is vital that you attempt and make it to the ideal location and train your own body to finally reach the absolutely balanced posture.

Later this pose, try out the forward bend present to excite the nervous system. Afterward it's possible to attempt the fish present, it strengthens the torso lungs and muscles.

Next pose is known as cobra pose. Women who have problems with degenerative issues might try out the cobra present, it arouses the pelvic and lower abdominal region, improving the flow and massaging the body organs.

Should you want to reinforce the back, then you definitely need to try out the locust pose. Locust pose is known to help prevent constipation.

The bow is just still another present to assist your spine area stay powerful and flexible at precisely the exact same period along with abdominal fat my additionally be reduced when the proper diet is put on. Furthering this yoga practice you are able to try out the half twist pose for the spines.

Breathing is an extremely essential aspect in practicing

yoga. You're able to learn appropriate method of breathing and enhance it by practicing exactly the crow pose. With this particular present, you are able to better your arm and joints stamina too. Afterward it is possible to try out the hands to foot pose and also the triangle. This pose necessitates the strength and flexibility.

At the end of most of these yoga exercise exercises; be certain you do the corpse present to recover any energy that's been lost throughout these totally free yoga practice also to offer rest to the entire body.

You are able to decide to try these completely free yoga exercises by one and watch for yourself that one's work the right for you personally. Knowing the poses which benefit you, only ensure you usually do not over stretch yourself into doing those exercises also that you observe exactly the exact same pair of exercises regularly.

Should you are considering taking a sort of practice with the purpose of creating yourself feel and look far better that you have to give very serious thought to yoga .

Yoga works in your human body and mind and its results is understood in lots of diverse aspects - within our own bodies, their own health insurance and the way they look, and on our heads - how we view the planet.

Therefore, just how do yoga exercises change from other kinds of exercise?

Yoga exercises, also called asanas or postures, are put on the full body of the body. Alternatively,

Lots of other workout regimes really are a sort of

technology placed on the muscles of their human body. Which usually means that yoga exercises are more worried about more than simply the shallow growth of muscles. The bearings utilized in yoga exercises have a tendency to normalize the purposes of the full organism.

The advantage of yoga exercises is they could modulate the involuntary processes of respiration and help the flow and digestion, elimination and metabolism etc. The exercises also function to impact the working of the glands and glands, in addition to the nervous system and also your head. This outcome is reached by doing heavy breathing as your system is put into a variety of postures. Every one of those yoga exercises creates an alternative totality from the connection that is functional inside the organism.

Thus, yoga can influence person physically, emotionally, morally and emotionally. Yoga highlights the doctrine of exercise. Under its training experiences a feeling of awakening. Each one's abilities are more heightened, and yet one accomplishes equilibrium and endurance through these aerobic exercises, some of which are modeled following the movements of different

Creatures. In aerobic exercises, comfort is educated as a art, breathing for being a science, and emotional control of your human body for a way of harmonizing the body, mind, and soul.

The advanced stages of yoga require several years of special preparation-practices. Now's manner of living, its pace and environment, imply this is tricky to realize. But, practicing yoga, yoga and heavy breathing and relaxation methods, with some of the period dedicated to meditation and concentration is some thing

Everyone could reach.

Yoga exercises may have a beneficial impact on those that suffer from illness or disease. Whilst it isn't ready to cure those matters, practicing yoga may implies that obstacles and impurities have been removed to ensure nature may do its curative work.

Therefore, if you're searching for a sort of exercise is effective favorably on your system and mind, and also something which is relatively simple to squeeze in to a daily routine then not consume exercises. The expanding prevalence of yoga exercises ensures you will likely locate a yoga center or some gymnasium that provides local classes in your town. If, nevertheless, you don't need enough time for you to attend classes you'll find lots of novels and dvd's on aerobic exercises, which means that you may perform it in your home at some period if it's suitable for you personally.

Within just a day or two of performing yoga exercises it's likely to come to feel revitalized as well as healthier. Continued training of yoga exercises may make us fitter and more joyful.

The ideal in Indian conventional kind of exercising is meditation that can supply a helpful way by that to boost your brain and the soul within and adds essential strength to your individual's human body and it all needs to gain from yoga will be really to master about the appropriate bearings in addition to methods of breathing. Ostensibly, everyone may do yoga practice provided that they have a very yoga mat and also actually, should they ensure selecting the suitable yoga mat, then they also are able to enjoy greater and a lot more comfortable at the exact same time as relaxing cycling practice.

Earlier you choose a particular yoga practice mat tote it pays to you to have a look at the different available yoga exercises mats and also the truth is, choosing a eco-yoga physical exercise mat is likely to soon be wise since the one that's surely built from pvc will place your health in danger and so needs to be avoided because a wonderful bargain as you possibly can.

One in the accessories that are essential to save your mat is truly a yoga mat tote which also helps you take your yoga mat together with you where you move. In reality, the better yoga mats could be folded along with wrapped and those are able to be placed within a yoga mat tote and performed with you too as useful for keeping your yoga exercises mat whilst it isn't being used.

An excellent yoga mat tote should be capable of carrying out a significant yoga mat which can measure up to hundred inches and additionally the yoga mat tote is good fitted to carrying along on your own journeys plus in addition, it helps assure the mat remains comfy and is protected from the weather and naturally, out of dirt.

You are able to find quite a-few diverse styles from which to choose if it concerns a superb yoga mat tote and the one which you opt for will be dependent on the size at precisely the exact same period as fabric employed and depends upon its layouts and you'll discover also various models for you to elect choose pick from. The simple truth isthat it's rather typical to run into that yoga practice mat totes are made from silk and sometimes cotton whereas people manufactured out of jute as well as oftentimes velvet may also be rather well-known.

You want to create sure the yoga exercises mat tote that you want on buying is lasting plus it needs to be hardy enough to resist normal damage and in addition, it might likewise encourage to have a very yoga mat tote that's watertight, also for everyone these features, a handbag made from cotton will probably soon be most suitable.

If it concerns a yoga mat handbag constructed from lace or silk, they'll generally have cotton liner (thick) which contributes to their durability too as durability and several have very interesting patterns and comprise vibrant colors too as possess brilliant textures and are appropriate to people that need something out in your standard.

Yoga exercises would be the perfect way to spare your mind also to focus heavily. As soon as you've seen a stressful situation, the thoughts, body and soul is worn outside and exhausted. The reason of them may possibly have been out of the interaction with different people or something which have resulted in a pity, anger, melancholy and disappointment in you personally. These feelings generated out of those circumstances needs to be published so you may live a more joyful life. 1 effective method and also way expressing your own outpoured feelings and feelings is by simply doing yoga exercises. Once you truly feel like crying aloud or breaking the tv, you're able to as an alternative release your anxiety through yoga exercises which can be effective and beneficial. Such a plan has functioned in lots of ways for diverse men and women. People of us who do not find sufficient time for themselves may perform yoga exercises as a way to relieve themselves. Sometimes, work has captured us up so closely we do not find time for you to curl up and state ourselves. Yoga exercises are among the better remedies for this issue. Yoga exercises might also be implemented and heard from school. There are a number of sessions offering yoga clinics. The exercises you'll see in school might be performed in your home. In reality, you are able to learn a few yoga exercises in home by yourself. You are only going to need to desire a tv and a videotape. The tape reveals the following steps and steps for each yoga practice. Throughout a weary and heavy daytime, you also may set just a small commitment and time in doing aerobic exercises. Also bear in mind that in doing yoga, then you will have to be persistent in practicing the exercises in order it will soon take effect and you'll find over time developments in your own entire body. After doing the yoga exercises, then you ought to curl up for the consequence of those positions occur place. This way, your system will collect the outcomes. Before doing the yoga exercises, then you ought to lay at a relaxed posture which means that you may focus well and never be diverted by outside forces. You won't feel discomfort or pain too. Yoga exercises may be done anytime of the time provided that you're free. Even though it selects virtually no moment, still, the very best time to clinic it really is each daytime. Before eating your breakfast, then your mind is dependent upon its condition of calmness and clear of distractions. This really may be the best time to accomplish exercises. Before doing the exercises, make certain the heart is ready. It ought not feel any self or pain. It's crucial to maintain a fantastic center which means your brain can get the job done well. The right spot to accomplish your yoga exercises would be a silent location. It ought to be well ventilated and free of most of disagreeable things as well as smell. You ought to be liberated of all probable distractions. Keeping a fantastic tummy can be crucial therefore you may feel well along with your gastrointestinal tract answers accurately. What you ought to do is to drain your intestines and clean your noses. You ought to stay fit and clean. Now you have obviously understood the critical reminders, then you can begin your yoga exercises and work out your way.

Yoga is among the exercises which have boundless health and fitness benefits; by the robust and elastic body, a calm mind, a luminous beautiful skin, fat reduction for healing. It gives immense benefits which not only joins your system, but additionally boosts your head in addition to the breathing strategy. It compels stability and leaves your life more serene, happier and fulfilling.

Routine yoga training will give you with all around fitness center. This suggests you won't you should be getting physically healthy; however you'll also be receiving mentally and mentally fit throughout the exercises. That is authorized by different exercises such as positions, breathing methods and meditation which yoga comprises.

Now you can even shed weight with yoga in the event that you're too heavy or in the event that you only need to drop some weight to better the physique. Once you take out yoga clinics, you'll begin becoming sensitive regarding the foods which you will likely be giving your entire body and the perfect time you'll be carrying foods. While doing so, you'll be keeping tabs on your own weight reduction.

Yoga methods can allow you to relieve stress that collects daily. With only a couple of minutes of yoga, then you will really feel liberated on the own body in addition to mind from some other stress which you may be going right through. The yoga poses, meditation and also the breathing processes can assist you to overcome tension and melancholy. In an advanced level yoga grade, it is possible to even utilize yoga exercises to detoxing your system and de-stressing mind.

Still another health advantage you can receive from yoga exercises will be inner peace. When a few folks desire inner serenity, they see quite places rich in natural magnificence. Nonetheless, it's also great to be aware you could experience inner peace anywhere you might be and in any given moment. As an example, doing yoga exercises on your house will be able to assist you to get the inner peace that's available right in it. You do not necessarily need to attend a particular spot to have it. Inner-peace is quite essential in calming a troubled mind.

Now you may also gain from improved resistance if you execute routine exercises. For the body to get the job done well, your bodymind and soul require to blend together. When there was an irregularity within your system, your head is going to be influenced inducing to experience guilt or unpleasantness. The yoga poses can also enable you to strengthen your muscles and also massage your own muscles. Besides relieving you in stress, breathing and meditation techniques may even enhance your own immunity.

Routine Pilates exercises can make the own body to own better posture and flexibility. Should you really miss a human body that's strong, flexible and supple, the trick is to add yoga in your ordinary routine. The own body tissues will be elongated and tone plus they'll become stronger. The own body posture once you stand, sit, sleep or walk will probably be made better. In the event that you will often possess human body aches because of incorrect position, yoga methods may assist you to overcome them.

Now you may likewise feel pumped up with energy in the event you maintain routine exercises. Should you feel tired out by the ending of your afternoon, or you also detect taking out multiple activities to become quite tiring, a couple minutes of exercising every day will make you feeling lively and fresh daily. Throughout your afternoon, you'll likely be refreshed and prepared to execute those activities of daily.

When you execute yoga exercises frequently, and you will establish greater intuition. Meditation can enhance your instinctive capability and permit one to comprehend cheaply what ought to be achieved, how it has to be achieved and exactly what period it has to be carried out. This can allow you to yield very good outcomes or boost your performance in your everyday pursuits.

In early India, yoga has been a method of living that comprised moral, moral, religious, and physiological components. Postures (asana) were also an essential, but tiny sector of the early clinic. Today, a lot of men and women make use of the word "yoga" to mean a certain sort of physical exercise, even while being totally oblivious of its own spiritual part, making the present-day model of meditation a shadow of its former self. Some classes wind without a time spent from the worthiness of pranayama, relaxation, or meditation.

To put it yet another way, the vital yoga mat, utilized in today's exercise variant, could just be needed to get a modest part of a genuine yoga clinic. As stated by maharishi Patanjali's writings, at the yoga sutras, asana is simply among eight limbs over yogic philosophy - most which can be utilized to organize for the greatest marriage of someone's inner intellect together with worldwide comprehension. As stated by proponents of conventional yoga, it's not possible to accomplish enlightenment simply by doing a bodily practice, even when a person practices the very complex postures.

In addition to providing a twisted view of this original clinic, contemporary yoga was sidetracked and used as a procedure to market popularity and sell pictures to people. This consists of personal stardom, and any such thing from correct organic mats, for high priced high style accessories and clothing. While this isn't inherently bad whatsoever, it scarcely looks like the humble way of life, and unwavering dedication, of those numerous sages, who retained yoga living for generations throughout Sanskrit texts and oral teachings. When yogic teachings gained worldwide awareness, it was just natural to modern yoga to simply take its own individuality.

This doesn't follow that the bodily exercises at modern meditation are poor or some less efficient compared to people at different tasks. In reality, asanas and leaks maybe more powerful than a number of different sorts of exercise. Studies have revealed that yoga movement improves physical health and fitness, help prevent illness, reduce depression and stress, reduce anxiety, promote comfort, and an overall awareness of wellbeing. Purists, however, could wonder if these fitness-based styles ought to really be called yoga.

The fact remains that few folks in the 21stcentury, are most likely to devote long intervals at ashrams because apprentices, meditating, and living the life span of some conventional yogi. In reality, a little bit of yoga is definitely greater than no yoga in any way. If modern yoga exercises is really helping create a more healthy and more peaceful society, also reducing the amazing price of health care bills, it's magic in itself.

Still another issue with modern yoga is that the significantly confusing actuality that a few folks think it to be counterproductive with their own religious beliefs or opinion systems. Meditation is a life style, not just a religion. Yoga doesn't discriminate. It will not look to hinder human beliefs or rationale, and anybody is welcome to appreciate its benefits. Afterall, who can assert with a fitter, happier, more peaceful planet?

The exercise is imagined to loosen the central nervous system and also stabilize the whole human body, mind, and soul. It's thought with its own enthusiasts to steer clear of certain ailments. Doing this type of exercise usually help make the human body's immune mechanisms strong assisting your own body to be in a position to manage lots of disorders like annoyance, fatigue and so forth. The curative rate of a personal accident or only a wound can be additionally enhanced. In addition, yoga practice was employed to lessen hyper tension degrees, reduce stress, and boost coordination, endurance, attention, sleeping, and food digestion. Medical professionals along with scientists have been researching latest the huge benefits of exercising regularly. Studies demonstrate that it might potentially decrease the signs of many popular and sometimes life-threatening disorders including arthritis, arteriosclerosis, acute fatigue, diabetes, obesity, aids, asthma attack along with weight loss issues.

Together with treating disorders, yoga practice is presently one among the choices for drugs. Together with yoga exercises like a combination of physical exercises, breathing exercises, and meditation, it turns to a especially effective type of physical activity for people that have certain medical difficulties. For anyone who have cardiovascular disease, various studies have proven yoga practice to aid people young and old. In particular, the exercise appears to enhance cardiovascular disease in lots of ways, including controlling elevated blood pressure rates and increasing immunity to emotional stress. Scientific tests made at yoga establishments in India have recorded impressive success in relieving asthma. Additionally, it has been proven that asthma conditions can normally be prevented by way of yoga courses without turning into medicinal drugs. Yoga can be thought to decrease pain by helping the brain's pain center regulates the gate-controlling system found in the back and also the release of natural pain killers in the physique. Cardiovascular exercises utilized in yoga additionally can reduce strain. Considering the fact that muscles have a tendency to curl up once you breathe, widening time of exhalation can help provide comfort decreasing strain. Recognizing breathing helps to acquire calmer, less fast respiration and help with comfort and pain control. Yoga has got the chance to buffer against the damaging impact of physiological self-objectification also to build up embodiment and wellbeing.

Moreover, the practice was broadly studied as a way in lowering (and occasionally remove) many cardiovascular risks. A number of these unwanted side effects include lower the circulation of blood, renal system failure, menopausal failure, as well as blindness. Many researchers believe practicing yoga and with daily aid services and products on a frequent basis might help stimulate blood circulation and massage tissues, which regularly can offer long-term bodily advantages to people fighting diabetes. In addition, the practice of yoga may provide long-term benefits for those who have diabetes because this was ascertained to decrease sugar levels, obtaining a fantastic result on every kind of diabetes, including type 1 and type 2 diabetes.

Yoga exercise is actually the very best medicine for several sort of health issues and also a very excellent refresher of individual brain, body and soul. It helps to get a person emotionally and emotionally productive. Consequently, everyone should start performing yoga exercise often to remain healthy and fit to very existence.

CHAPTER SIX

❧

Sciatica exercises for pain management

S ciatica anxiety can be tricky to live with, impacting every part of a sufferer's daily life. There are lots of alternatives for sciatica pain alleviation; it could be handled by inpatient home remedies, such as cold and hot therapy and physical exercise. Sciatica pain may be handled using drugs. In acute circumstances, pain may be relieved or handled using operation.

In the last, bed remainder was frequently suggested for patients suffering from pain. Nowadays, however, doctors and physical therapists equally are counseling against this clinic. As an alternative, a normal gentle exercise regime is advised. Targeted stretches, such as yoga methods, are also utilized to alleviate pain. Sciatica treatment may be gotten with cold and hot therapy in your home. Applying ice packs to the affected area offers treatment. Filled with warmth provides the muscles that are affected an opportunity to relaxand relieving strain over the compressed nerve and also relieving the pain that the victim feels.

Drug can be also a choice for sciatica pain alleviation. Sciatica pain is treated using a anti inflammatory medication like ibuprofen or codeine. In acute instances, cortisone shots might also be managed for temporary treatment. Sufferers must remember, nevertheless, why these drugs simply alleviate the annoyance. They usually do not heal the underlying problem.

In acute instances, sciatica sufferers may buy respite from operation. If puberty is being brought on by a spinal trauma, like a slipped or herniated disc, surgery may alleviate the rear harm, and so the stress on the sciatic nerve. If you're having chronic gastrointestinal pain, then speak with your physician about what options may be ideal for you personally.

The best way can lyrica and sciatica link solely to another? Anxiety with sciatica can impair the usual lifetime and cause agonizing pain. It could and can restrict your ability to walk and the skill to proceed. Usually the pain is principally using a single side of their human anatomy. It's going to begin at the back and then proceed its way down the cool and all of the way to the feet.

Additionally, it is frequently abbreviated because of disorder in reality, lyrica and endometriosis really are a combination which helps relieve the chronic pain which could be a consequence of the compressed or pinched nerve or a irritation to the nerves. The therapy needed would all depend on what's causing the pinched nerve.

Lyrica and sciatica pain control is an extremely significant part the nerve procedure process. Any movement will probably lead to pain, and also the patient chooses to confine their movement due to the pain entailed. If they simply sit that is a lot easier than most of the annoyance. However, this may be dangerous and will lead to stiffness in the joints and muscles. And also this can lead to more pain and problems.

The secret to handling so, the trick to all other remedies for sciatica would be really exercise. Pain management is essential, but even thus the affected individual is preferred to sustain an inpatient workout regime.

Sciatica pain control is just one of the main facts to take into consideration when treating your own pain. People all over the globe suffer with plantar pain and also a few understand just how to manage it. Below are a number of ways which you may safely and effortlessly maintain your sciatica symptoms off.

One method to deal with your sciatica is through exercises and stretches. Even though these are extremely effective, few folks would follow on an everyday basis. It's imperative that you stay together with stretching which will work and throw off the ones which aren't. Attempt to accomplish your exercises and stretches regular, even when it's only for five full minutes. After a month or two or weeks, then you will realize a dramatic decline in pain. But do not end there. Regular you ought to be continuously exercising or extending, even when pain has escalated. This will reduce the possibility of one's pain coming back and with you reside with sedation again.

Still another method to deal with your sciatic pain is via therapy. Seeing a physical therapist in an everyday basis can reduce your symptoms, sometimes the initial moment. Even though this is often frustrating, it's extremely powerful. Going to the community physician and advocating seeing a physical therapist can be the starting place. As soon as you've discovered the one that's ideal for you, stay to this app. Establish certain goals for yourself and stay motivated. The further you're inclined to triumph, the faster that your result will likely be.

As you're able to easily see, there really are an assortment of means to aid in managing your own sciatica. Make sure you sick with whichever application that you proceed through and stay motivated. The trick is copying, the longer you elongate or view a therapist, the greater your odds will be for a fast and effortless recovery.

In case you're feeling pain in your own lower back when you bend or stretch also it melts to your thighs, you then could be undergoing sciatica. However, what exactly is sciatica? It's a pain symptom that caused the aggravation of the sciatic nerve. The pain usually begins at the low back and could stretch to the foot and calf based upon the affected nerve origin. Sciatica isn't just a disease alone but a symptom caused the other health illness. Individuals who're often afflicted with sciatica are afflicted by the herniated disk. One other element which directly impacts aggravation and swelling in the sciatic nerve produces the signs of sciatica.

The sciatic nerve is the largest nerve in your system. Its neural roots run in the thoracic back located at the low back stretching throughout the buttocks, shoulders and lower limb. If this nerve becomes irritated or inflamed it produces pain which looks such as a leg . It generates sitting nor standing difficult on account of the high level of pain it soothes. An average of the pain is aggravated after sitting, coughing or sneezing. Illness in severe puberty usually lasts for four to eight weeks plus reduces on a unique based upon the causative agent.

Sciatica is frequently brought on by the slipping of disks. It's normal in people between the ages of 30-50 partially as a result of aging. The overall damage of the encompassing muscular of the spine can readily be afflicted with any abrupt pressure on the discs. The discs function as a pillow of this bone at the low spine of course, whether or not it deteriorates can lead into the manifestation of puberty; the high degree of pain caused by sciatica fluctuates.

The compression of the thoracic nerve contributes to sciatica. After the disk slips or lumps, pain in the back is the initial symptom which is being shown. Its symptoms can include tingling sensation, numbness and tingling sense.

Diagnosis of sciatica normally comprises a comprehensive clinical assessment. In general, the physician explains the way a pain started and its own symptoms. Appropriate knowledge and comprehension are crucial to your affected individual to clearly comprehend what's sciatica and just how can this affect them. Your health care provider could also need to examine its symptoms and signs through a concrete examination. Physical exam can also help determine its origin to be in a position to offer a definite outlook. The evaluation can be also utilized to pin point the most nerves that are affected. Other evaluations like Xray and mri could be recommended for additional evaluation.

Ostensibly the most important objective of treatment for sciatica would be always to diminish pain, stiffness and increase freedom. The cure for sedation would ordinarily involve rehab, medical and surgery direction. If puberty happens untreated it may possibly result in a chronic illness and further complications. Intense sciatica illness usually goes off with good time and rest, with no necessity for surgery or some other medical direction. There are means to help stop sciatica such as routine exercise to strengthen muscles and also maintaining appropriate body posture in any way times.

The lumbar nerve roots originate from the spine and at the time they're susceptible to impingement out of a disk prolapse, inducing compression or inflammation of the nerve and also the signs of sciatica. Sciatic leg pain isn't common, affecting 3 to 5 percent of adults along with both genders equally. Men tend to be more inclined to receive it inside their 40s and ladies in their 50s, together with pain symptoms lasting more than 6 weeks in up to a quarter of cases. Physiotherapists are routinely requested to oversee the administration of sciatica.

When the intervertebral disk material prolapses, it induces injury by 2 mechanisms: direct mechanical compression of this nerve and chemical aggravation. The disk material shouldn't be outside the disk and its particular toxic compounds help swelling the neural as well as its surrounding structures, leading to congestion of the flow and also of their guts's ordinary message conduction. As the prolapse accounts for that sciatica it hasn't yet been demonstrated that the larger the prolapse the more acute anyone's pain.

The fantastic forces that we inflict on the minimal back imply the thoracic intervertebral disks suffer structural alterations along with prolapses. Many tasks involve a substantial degree of grip, such as bending over, performing motions in a vertical posture and lifting the arms apart from your system. This greatly magnifies the forces onto the disks and because of their fluid mechanisms that they suffer 3 5 times the heaps on the manhood. This could create the disk walls to bluff, providing feeble locations and predisposing to prolapse at a while.

The onset of lumbosacral radiculopathy can be surprising with low backpain along with some other spine pain can disappear at the onset of leg pain. Worsening facets are coughing, coughing and sitting together with bending or taking a stand common easing facet. Sciatic pain generally happens from the buttock back or side of their calf and leg and to the foot. In case the disk prolapse is high up (prolapses at disk degrees 11 to 13 are 5 percent of their total) the pain could possibly take the front part of the thigh no more compared to the knee. An individual might have a isolated field of pain but have a prolapse.

The physiotherapist will choose the individual's history with special awareness of "warning flag" which are signs of a severe medical reason behind the spine pain and the affected person won't be suitable to get physio. Weight loss, fever, night sweats, age (under 20 or more 55), issues with bowel and bladder control, acute beyond health background and also nighttime pain is going to be noticed. Any doubt implies citizenship to a health care provider for analysis. The physio will see some postural abnormalities and also the disposition, activity and position response of these pain signs.

A patient with spinal radiculopathy might display strange posture, sometimes flexed forwards and not able to bend backward, with a one-piece trunk change. Physiotherapists assess the capacity to do spinal motions, any pattern of restriction or trend for the annoyance to centralize on perennial moves. Physios can examine the springs, sensibility and muscular capability to carry out the neural examination. This and also the right leg raising test allow the physio to assess which of their spinal nerves is very likely to be to blame.

Discogenic pain may vary with recurrent motions, dispersing further towards the leg in towards the spine, the latter being termed as centralization. Physiotherapists utilize this happening to diagnose and cure disk related spine pain and also analyze the joints of the thoracic as knee and thigh pain might be known in an osteoarthritic hip joint. The complete history and examination eliminate patients who want medical referral for analysis and permit the physio to make cure plan.

Physio therapy laughter remedies incorporate many remedies: manipulation, mobilization procedure, lumbar equilibrium, myofascial discharge, McKenzie procedure (especially beneficial in disk prolapse), stabilizing massage, massage and soft tissue methods, painkillers, instruction of the individual, information on the ideal position to alleviate extreme aching pain along with remainder. Sciatica hastens as the inflammation and pressure simplicity however physiotherapists might suggest a continuous exercise plan to keep up straight back wellness over the very long run.

Most people today suffer with several diverse sorts of back pain and related back injuries, for example sciatica. When in pain, we all know to do is search out solutions. Broadly speaking we count upon a family practitioner or local clinical practitioner who we now have learned. This starts the individual at the "medical model" way of a settlement with the problem. Alas, the final effect for this particular version is frequently operation. Operation, even though sometimes necessary, is rarely the most effective alternative for first-time patients using sciatica. From another article we'll go over the positive aspects of chiropractic care to operation. It's going to tackle the good and the negative for both sorts of treatment.

The study discussed here has been ran with the national spine center at Alberta Canada and released in October of 2010 at the journal of manipulative and physiological therapeutics [inch]. The control group consisted of 40 patients who had been struggling with sciatica for longer than a couple of weeks. These patient's undergone treatments using pain drugs, making life style alterations, withstood physical therapy, failed massage or acupuncture without the consequences. Whenever these processes failed to work; their chief physician referred them to specialists which deemed them appropriate candidates for operation.

The people within this category were split in to two classes: one group experienced a medical procedure identified as microdiscectomy and one other type has been treated with a chiropractic utilizing conventional procedures. The patients got the ability of experiencing one other kind of treatment after a couple of weeks when these weren't pleased with the very first therapy.

What were the consequences?

The two groups saw noticeable improvements over baseline scores - significance which they watched noticeable improvements where as previous approaches had neglected. The complete 60 percent of the study participants profited from chiropractic spinal manipulation to the exact same level as though they failed operation. After 12 months there wasn't any difference in effect success dependent on the procedure technique. Which usually means that the total 60 percent of people called operation by their own primary care physicians and recognized as surgical applicants by the neuro surgeon might actually become similar results with chiropractic care. That will be a whole lot of potentially unnecessary anesthesia, cutting and er period. There's 1 paragraph from the results section with this study that's not hard to overlook, but exceptionally crucial. There have been originally 120 applicants which 60 met the study criteria and were asked to participate. Of those 60, 20 refused. Why? Because they'd not been given a substitute for operation; including as spinal manipulation. They did not desire to take part in the study and also be placed in the operation group without trying the spinal column manipulation! That really is incredibly telling. Not only does this demonstrate that there's still a demand for people and primary care physicians to learn about more regarding chiropractic processes, but in addition, it shows that folks comprehend the risks and costs of operation and would like to exhaust other possibilities.

This was that the initial study to look at those who'd neglected conventional medical direction of sciatica. Now many patients which neglect 'conservative maintenance' are known for a surgical test. We understand that 60 percent of those individuals can avoid surgery and have similar long-term effects together with acupuncture.

Sciatica has come to be the most commonplace back pain syndrome which affected millions of those mature people across the entire world. Cure for sciatica involves just proper straight back pain control. Sciatica treatments have come to be a multi-billion industry due to the expanding amount of men and women experiencing back pain. Physicians, nurses and other pros have gained advantage over offering the very best possible plan of treatment for relieving sciatica.

Treatments for sciatica demand traditional and non-conventional procedures. But people are now actually beginning to adopt the notion of choosing unconventional across the traditional treatments. With the existing uncertainty offered by a poor world economy, the seek out some other kinds of calculations revealed a radical increase through recent years. People today would like to come across a much cheaper and efficient method to put a stop with their unending struggle with plantar pain.

Ordinarily, direction for sciatica doesn't require to elect for extreme measures like operation and drugs, and unless there's a demand for you. Conservative kinds of treatments are consistently the first line of cure for sciatica. But appropriate identification of this inherent spinal illness stays the very best & most prosperous treatment in combating its outward symptoms. That really is being highlighted since burnout is a generally abbreviated symptom and also the most reasons the plan of treatment employed proves for a collapse. If you're some of the men and women who've tried virtually every treatment potential but still without a success, then a prognosis of the chief reason for sciatica is most probably undervalued.

Complete mattress remainder has become easily the most conservative approach that's ordinarily suggested by physician for being a cure for sciatica. Patients have been counseled to take short-term bed fractures in order for that pain to subside. Long term childbirth and protracted hospitalization are definitely frustrated. Deficiency of movement and also in activity could inflict more damage as a result of development of muscular corrosion. If your doctor happens to information more and protracted periods of bedrest, may too think about another most suitable choice.

Alternative treatments like chiropractic clinics, acupuncture and acupuncture are found to be a good method of treating sciatica. It has treatments and clinics that are much different from the standard treatments. It's obviously led by a professional or specialist such as for instance a certified therapist, acupressure pro and acupuncturist. They're the men and women who commence the treatment to make certain it's correctly handled.

CHAPTER SEVEN

❦

What to expect from pain management?

People frequently wrongly think about treatment by way of a pain management specialist as comprising just narcotic "painkillers "

But, the custom of pain medicine or pain control is identification driven only as with other healthcare specialties. As goes to a cardiologist to get a test of cardiovascular illness and receives treatment primarily based on a exceptional identification, a call into your pain management pro ends in unique treatment as every patient having pain is likewise different. The subject of pain medicine can be involved with the prevention, diagnosis, analysis, treatment, and treatment of debilitating ailments.

Infection affects more Americans compared to diabetes, cardiovascular problems and cancer combined. You can find approximately 116 million Americans with chronic pain, defined as pain that has lasted longer than three weeks and 25 million people who have severe pain.

Just like other physicians, the pain control pro should assess each affected individual and generate a plan for treatment on the basis of the individual's symptoms, examination and other findings. As an instance, the cardiologist must first examine you personally and create a few determinations. These generally include deciding if a cardiovascular illness will respond to fat reduction and exercise, if you've got elevated blood pressure and also want medication to reduce your blood pressure or if your cholesterol is either raised or if you own a congestion and desire an enhancement procedure or as a final resource, if you may possibly have to get called a coronary artery for coronary bypass operation.

All patients with coronary problems do not require the exact medications. This is contingent on the origin of the issue. Just because there are various treatments out there for cardiovascular problems, you can find certainly a huge quantity of treatment alternatives out there for orthopedic pain.

Even though patients may proceed into a pain management doctor because they "hurt," as they visit a cardiologist since all of them have heart issues, all pain doesn't reply to narcotics. It's a unfortunate and common offender when patients head to the pain management physician, they'll soon be treated with narcotics.

Treatments for spinal or spinal pain change like treatments for cardiovascular infection vary. It is dependent upon what's your explanation for your trouble.

First importantly, it's necessary to see there are several kinds of spinal or sinus pain. An individual may have muscle soreness, ligamentous pain, joint pain, bone pain, and distress as a result of herniated discs, pain by a fracture pain or pain by a pinched nerve or a nerve injury. Anxiety drugs are prescribed in relation to the resource of the painkillers.

Some patients that arrived at pain control never require

pain medications. They can answer a ultrasound, additional intervention, bracing, or even into physical therapy. Our knowledge has grown into where we now know more how lousy posture and walking all perpetuate emotional pain. With complex utilization of exercises, tailored into someone's particulars demands, physical therapy could be helpful.

An test in physical therapy may possibly show that the individual's pain is due to lousy movement, tight muscles, rigid muscles, feeble musculature, or postural issues. As an instance, we are aware that patients with degenerative disc disorder, where the disc between 2 bones has begun to tear and wear, can reduce the pressure in the disc by exercising to boost your heart musculature and reduce or eliminate backpain.

Just like that the cardiologist who plays interventional procedures like coronary artery catheterizations, pain control physicians perform interventional approaches to reduce or eliminate pain, and operation as in different regions of medicine must be the final holiday season.

When you originally goto a cardiologist as a result of slight problem, i will be confident that a large part of you wouldn't ask"do i want surgery?" one wants to research different options before surgical interventions have been researched.

Out of experience, I've learned that patients perform best with treatment using way of a pain management specialist should they encounter with the exact same open mind and mindset at which they have been prepared to research a lot of options and become focused primarily on becoming narcotics or believing that operation is their sole alternative.

I used the illustration of this cardiologist because i understand that a large part folks might like that the cardiologist research all options before speaking us to a coronary artery. This is exactly the exact approach this someone ought to use while they've an ill or spinal issue. Always inquire about nonsurgical alternatives for the spinal or esophageal pain.

The pain management doctor, just like the cardiologist, doesn't function operation. Even the cardiologist does interventional methods, related medications, also manages your cardiac rehabilitation plan. Like wise a pain management doctor manages and sends your physical therapy or rehab application, prescribes medications, also plays interventional procedures. The two cardiologist and pain practitioner will probably consult with a physician if required.

Timing is essential to the results of one's treatment. You ought not delay a test for cardiovascular problems, nor if you proceed to discount spinal or spinal pain, and then wait overly long before trying a test having a pain specialist. I've seen too many patients wait too late during their treatment before looking for a pain specialist. As with other specialties, premature intervention could result in a better result.

Infection direction is a practice. It is made of numerous treatment plans and much more to the point, the remedy to the pain might well not be exactly the exact same since it really is for your own neighbor. Exactly enjoy a pacemaker could be the procedure of choice for the better half but maybe not the treating choice for you personally once you find that a cardiologist.

Innovations in pain-management

There has really been a wonderful shift in the life style of people who are in today's period, and people who have grown to be more prone to disease and illness. Anxiety is just one of those severe health problems that a lot of ailing men and women have. Anxiety can be painful, while it's actually a minor trauma or perhaps a life-threatening disease. There really are a range of trusted practices in U.S. who have produced innovative practices and remedies in managing pain. The indicators of pain could be alleviated with medications; however, medications have any unwanted effects. The growth and progress in technology have given rise to the invention of high level techniques and medications. The indicators of pain differ from one individual to another. It's dependent upon the individual's age, sex and physical stature. By working closely with the individual patient, a physician and pharmacist may prepare the suitable dose strength for extreme pain control.

Managing pain with drugs

Recognizing the idea of pain and its own control methods are shifting constantly. Various brand-new therapy plans are be-ings researched and introduced on an everyday basis. The most recent creations within the specialty of pain control would be of terrific value to the physicians in addition to professionals. A number of the qualities of latest processes contain achieving safe and durable relief systems that treat all sorts of human body aches. A number of the usual kinds of pains contain back pain, muscular, pain and pains related to illness or disease. For the majority of those pains, opioids having a prescription are regarded as effective on a momentary basis. Nevertheless, the opioid might decrease tolerance levels and also have any negative effects. Additionally, there are anti inflammatory and anti-inflammatory medications that have different negative effects, but are somewhat less habitforming.

Managing pain with remedies

There has become a excellent development in the specialty of pain control during treatments. Some of those advanced remedies that handle pain comprise celerel, painawaypro and therapize. These remedies expel the demand for narcotics. These treatments are utilized to take care of all types of pains which have neck pain back pain, postop pain and skin care conditions. The advanced remedies assist the individual in treating muscle strain in a simple way, regaining in less time, and increasing muscular strength.

Alternative pain management remedies

Additional studies have shown that conventional herbs may sometimes possess a long-term constructive effect, especially on arthritic painkillers. Included in these are the ingestion utilization of essential oils. Many essential oils possess pain and anti-inflammatory reducing properties if used frequently within a long-term using fewer side effects compared to many medication remedies. Consulting a naturopathic physician in combination with your doctor is preferred.

The two severe and chronic pain may interrupt your everyday living, especially with your leisure and work tasks. Perhaps this reason for pain is diagnosed or not, pain control methods may still help lots of people to no more suffer out of their ailment. In addition, it might permit the person to keep with their everyday tasks easily.

Infection is now turning into a significant problem within our society. In fact, nearly one third of the populace is afflicted by pain. Any pain is just one of the principal explanations for why individuals will proceed for appointment with their physician. Anxiety is a principal symptom in a lot of health circumstances, interfering with the standard of living and general functioning. If you're having pain on the human own body, don't just ignore it, thinking it will only go off. You won't ever know exactly what it's and it may just become worse should not assessed by your physician. This is the reason why pain control is a vital part of health since individuals forced to keep with the pain have a tendency to become miserable or using bad treatment benefits.

Earlier the ideal pain treatment therapy is given, health practitioners will determine the reason and also the kind of pain. Mild pain essentially does occur immediately and may be mild or acute. However, it typically lasts just a brief moment. On the flip side, chronic pain is much more disagreeable and also the pain may endure during a long time period, hence impacting day to day living. Individuals afflicted by pain may experience an extremely thorough evaluation which includes their health background so the health care provider can completely understand the status and apply the ideal pain control treatment and technique.

Specialists on pain control utilize various kinds of processes which may efficiently suppress and minimize the disagreeable sensation. There are quite a few facets which can be considered ahead of the ideal pain control is provided. It features the spot where pain is situated, era of the average person, amount of physical limit and seriousness of pain.

Now, with the progress within the sphere of health, pain control techniques also have improved. The analyzed and recognized pain control methods comprise medications, injections, physical and rehabilitative services, disk compression, electric therapy treatment, back stimulation, neural racking processes and even comfort methods. Please be aware the patient ought to have a dynamic role in working together with health-related conditions as a way to relish long-term respite from pain. Besides that, behavioral interventions may radically enhance the life span of their individual, thereby reducing the recurrence of pain.

Infection is a symptom brought on by physical, emotional, or emotional injury or disease. At a certain point over time you should have observed pain no one understand that nobody is afflicted by afflicted disorders. You're a individual and everybody else you understand the very last time you've assessed and hence are vulnerable to annoyance. As this is actually the situation, you then must discover to take care of pain therefore you're able to alleviate the symptom to some bearable situation for a damaging patient or individual. That really is the pain control is about and also you also do not have to be described as a healthcare personnel to become in a position to handle pain to get some body. Even though some assert that working with anxiety is limited just to the physiological part, you should understand that helping some body may also enhance their emotional and psychological expectancy once they understand some one is taking care of them.

Caring is a part of human character so we'll spend money on your own normal tendency to nurture someone else in doing pain direction therefore you will possess the confidence to simply help someone minimize his bodily injury. You have to continue to keep this in mind whenever you're doing pain control in order for the patient is going to learn that you're attempting to help them whatsoever and they'll perform their job too. You have to have your head set your patient may get rude, irritable, and also repulsive of one's service however, you need to know they are simply byproducts of these pain and so they aren't personal in character. Taking good care of annoyance additionally involves a whole lot of emotional and mental efforts to help that you are equipped for the hard function as provider of pain control.

There are many sorts of aches one individual might consume therefore many procedures are hailed for various treatments for your pain. Bear in mind you can't really get rid of the foundation of physical strain but can only relieve it into pain control. You're fixing the symptoms rather than the true source of annoyance. There are lots of procedures for overall pain control and it'll soon be discussed briefly below. As a first rule, some pain felt from means of physician ought to be consulted together with his doctor or physician so you realize the reason for the vexation and you're able to assist the individual more efficiently.

Analgesics or medication made to help in alleviating pain are available in many varieties but caution medication needs to be observed. Medicine built to alleviate pain ought to be given at a pain squat, as advocated by who (world health organization). Pain ladder is traditionally employed as an overall principle in supplying drug for any kind of pain - this explains that the degree of pain and which sort of medicine is ideal for the problem. Mild pain ought to be treated with paracetamol or aspirin. Mild to moderate pain necessitates paracetamol having a combination with hydrocodone turns out to be a lot more effective. Moderate to severe pain is normally treated with more serious drugs such as morphine and identical medications with care because of their addictive side effects. Physical approach in relieving pain comes with acupuncture, tens (transcutaneous electric nerve stimulation) and physiatry. The majority of these procedures apply physical rehab and drugs. Bipolar strategy is based on emotional processes such as behavioral and cognitive therapy, biofeedback, and hypnosis to alleviate anxiety from emotional intervention.

Infection direction is 1 field of medicine that includes found several technological advancements all over the world. Spurred with this world wide phenomenon, chronic pain control practices in developing countries also have begun using innovative methods from the regions of pain killers, pain assessment, and intervention for chronic pain control.

Chronic pain may consult with any form of pain which suffers even with a personal accident was treated, pain associated with some degenerative or persistent disorder, long-term pain for the cause can't be diagnosed, or cancer disorder. Generally, pain which lasts even with half a year is chronic and takes treatment.

The identification and treatment of a specific patient in a chronic pain management practice usually demands the participation of several specialists including anesthesiologists, psychiatrists, physiatrists, neurologists, along with physicians and nurses. Several treatments are combined in sequence to make the individual feel comfortable when the pain can't be ceased, to help him/her come back to work, to get rid of their depression, and also to boost their bodily operation. Ergo, these remedies are drugs, operation, emotional counseling, therapies to excite the nerves, life style shifts, anesthesiologic treatments, and rehab.

Drug advocated for patients in chronic pain control practices may alter out of maids for pain that's not so awful to narcotic medication for more acute pain. Physical therapy is just one common therapeutic technique employed in the administration of chronic illness such practices. It involves training the affected person to boost his flexibility, endurance, endurance and potency; to relocate a means which is structurally safe and appropriate; & above all to manage pain. Therapeutic exercise can be a significant quality of physical therapy.

Still another crucial technique employed in chronic pain management practices is transcutaneous electric nerve stimulation (tens). This method offers aid to patients suffering from conditions like back pain or pain at the back, by the usage of non invasive household energy.

To amount up, once pain has been chronic, entire freedom from the pain will be not difficult. But, chronic pain control practices, throughout the usage of multiple methods utilized together with one another, helps sufferers of chronic pain like a fitter and more energetic lifestyle.

Infection management physicians ordinarily chance to be

more anesthesiologists. Anesthesiologists make certain you're secure, weatherproof and comfortable throughout and after operation. Also they are at the office at the labour and delivery field, or at doctors' chambers at which debilitating tests or procedures have been performed. However, the processes employed by anesthesiologists have traveled outside these lands that are recognizable, also contributed to the evolution of a brand new kind of medicine called pain medication.

In many scenarios, an anesthesiologist directs a group of different physicians and specialists working together to ease your pain. The anesthesiologist or alternative pain medication physicians such as neurologists, oncologists, orthopedists, physiatrists and psychiatrists, and non-physician pros for example nurses, nurse practitioners, physician assistants, physical or rehab therapists and therapists, combine together to assess your problem. After an exhaustive appraisal, this group of pros develops a treatment plan for you personally.

Infection management physicians are pros at diagnosing the causes of the own pain in addition to curing the pain. Arthritis back and neck pain, cancer, pain, heart problems, migraines, shingles, along with phantom limb pain because of amputees are being among the most prevalent pain issues they generally manage.

Infection management physicians also treat severe pain brought on by operation, a painful disorder or even a significant accident. One of such pains is article knee joint replacement pain, headache during retrieval in the car collision, pain after chest or stomach operation, or pain related to sickle cell disorder. They could see to the patient at the clinic or at a hospital clinic.

The pain medication physician usually works closely together with your physician. They'll examine your medical records along with xrays as required. To get a very clear comprehension of the instance, they are going to provide you a thorough questionnaire. Your answers will enable them to assess the way your pain affects your everyday life. Pain management doctors may even perform a comprehensive physical exam on you personally. They could even select additional evaluations and examine all of the outcome to get the main cause of one's pain and also determine the way the situation may be solved.

No one likes to suffer with pain. A distressing sensation, pain can be really a result of the human anatomy to physical disease, trauma, or emotional illness. Pain is usually split into two types: acute and chronic. The former does occur unexpectedly as a result of trauma suffered by means of a tissue. The injury might be levied by whatever impacts human anatomy, i.e., operation, cancer or injury. Heartbeat and blood pressure usually increase in severe pain. However, when the reason for the pain is expunged, the pain normally goes off. Chronic pain, usually connected to some chronic illness, lasts more and there's a clear origin. Chronic lower back pain, chronic headaches, or cancer belongs to the category.

A pain management approach usually is contingent upon the character of this pain, i.e., if it's severe or chronic. Anxiety is usually handled by employing medical procedures, emotional procedures or other therapy approaches. In the instance of short-term severe pain due to an injury, normal medicines available on the counter, natural or herbal remedies and other medicines may be properly used. Chronic pain is much more difficult to handle, since it lasts longer and is much more technical.

Medi cal approaches might be broken to two chief techniques: medication treatment and operative intervention. Analgesic drugs may diminish or eliminate pain without affecting consciousness. Psychotropic drugs act in the mind, affecting the individual's psychological condition. An individual should, nevertheless, be careful in their long-term consequences. Still another procedure used is neural wracking, in that a medication is injected round the proper guts to protect against the pain from reaching the mind.

The reason for the surgical branch of neural pathways is the fact that should the pathway has been cracked the pain cannot undergo. Even though maybe not operative at the authentic sense, transcutaneous electric nerve stimulation (tens) arouses skin area across the site of this pain together with the assistance of a power stimulator, also simplifies the aggravation messages using a tingling sensation.

Anybody, who's working with long-term or intense pain, also knows the "pain" from this illness. Typically, patients spend a significant period of time together with primary care health practitioners, physical therapist, and also pros, expecting to obtain a more permanent alternative. Interventional pain control is actually a practical alternative in such circumstances, where the patient has tried the other treatment choices.

Recognizing interventional pain control

Interventional pain management can be a technical field in medicine that addresses the identification and treatment for long-term or severe pain along with other associated disorders. This really is more of a "multidisciplinary" system, that will be extended by a group of experienced doctors and caregivers. With interventional pain control, medical PR actioners make an effort to reduce chronic and acute pain, besides emphasizing better living. The therapy is completely distinct from other kinds of pain control since there's not any direct dependence on pain-relief medications. Typically, your doctor may refer the issue to your pain management physician, who'll choose the degree of treatment, based upon the truth of this situation. In the event there is interventional pain control, pain management doctor will come with physicians, physical therapists, occupational therapists, therapists, neurologist, and orthopedic physician as needed to take care of the condition through the use of minimally invasive procedures like epidural injections, facet blocks, trigger point injections, etc.

Matters worth understanding

Interventional pain control is very good for patients that suffer from back and neck pain. Physicians can utilize more than 1 approach into the illness, based upon the identification. Using steroidal shots at the joints and also epidural space is quite common, whereas shots are also utilized to deal with a spinal nerve root, and this is recognized as the supply of annoyance killers. Branch cubes are also useful for diagnostic intention accompanied closely by radio frequency ablation, while health practitioners might also utilize extra shots from the side joints. Discography can be employed to obtain the potential source of pain, also within this particular procedure, a special dye can be employed within an injectable shape to some disk to know the pathology better.

In a few scenarios, minimally-invasive procedures such as"radio frequency ablation" could be properly used for its healthcare divisions, in order to confine the movement of nuisance signs. Doctors can also indicate using heated electrodes for many nerves which take the pain signs, which procedure can be understood as rhizotomy. Maybe not to forget, physical therapy and other kinds of occupational treatments are also employed for your own procedure. Doctors also indicate life style changes to patients, even should they find some other expectation to get much better health.

Along with as the health society is getting more keenly conscious of the issue, physicians are thinking of regretting them. Therefore, a individual who has chronic back pain suffers, unless, their physician gets got the capability to refer these into a pain management center.

Referrals to a pain control Centre can be drawn up by almost any healthcare provider or an expert like a rheumatologist. Can this your physician passing the dollar because they don't really desire to bargain with you?

Perhaps not at all! If much of your maintenance or rheumatologist identifies one to a pain management center, it's in your own very best interest. A facility that's installed as interdisciplinary center, typically connected with hospitals or have an association with a medical college will have the ability to help handle your pain - free of restricted or no medicine

Because they truly are generally related to a hospital, so you can find medications like pain narcotics out there. However, they are going to initially make an effort to discover methods to handle your pain with no. What experts in those centers are finding is that too frequently, narcotics such as painkillers can give rise to a bunch of different issues.

The best way does all these facilities help?

Now you will be delegated to a group of pros. They'll examine the records that your main attention or rheumatologist sends them and they then are going to perform their very own preliminary assessments and analyzing. This might include blood workout, mris, x rays, etc.

Later they've this information gathered, the team will examine it and keep in touch with you regarding your history. What remedies or therapy you experienced and also how they worked or did not get the job done. You ought to be entirely fair and open with them around any portion of one's health history along with the way you live.

They will subsequently talk about this among themselves and generate a new plan which will be dealt with through the pain control center. You will assign to your chiropractor or physical therapist. You may possibly have meetings having a physiologist or psychologist. The team might believe you might take advantage of the massage therapist.

The goal of a pain control centre would be to exhaust other methods for managing the pain without narcotics. Sometimes, there'll be several medications prescribed in really tiny doses to get a while to workin combination with another remedies or remedies.

Exactly why the hesitation of medications?

A pain control center is dependent on what search has found. And research studies have discovered that people actually will undergo a rise in pain once they're on narcotics. Medication can alter how the body's immune system works. Endorphins are the organic painkiller. Granted there are people who are able to and can gain from narcotics, however also to automatically assume this could be the sole means to take care of pain would be an error.

Narcotic analgesics and opioids are very addictive to a patient. And there's also the concern of their interaction with other medications. For the ra patient, opioids won't cure their inflammation and also to get patients with fibromyalgia along with also the wide spread annoyance which is sold with, opioids just make it worse.

Later any operation, pain control is going to soon be important for both you and your physician. And if there's a degree of pain and distress to be likely after any sort of operation, your health care provider will require preventative measures to supply your ways to handle your pain. This is not just to continue to keep you comfortable, but if the own body is in distress, it cannot heal as fast as it will.

When you're just about to have surgery, your health care provider will go on your present medical wellbeing in addition to your health background. Always be fair and also notify them of any sort of medication you're taking, especially if you're already taking drugs to managing your own pain.

The kinds of pain to anticipate

Later operation, you might experience pain in regions which are going to be described as a surprise. Often times it's perhaps not at the operation website. Some regions where you may experience distress or pain following operation are:

- muscles - you might feel pain or distress in the field of one's spine, torso, chest, or shoulders. This stems from lying in 1 position on the table or the "tackling" the team may possibly perform together with you personally while at operation.
- throat - your neck may feel scratchy or tender. That really is from using any vibrations on your neck or mouth. Movement - any movement such as sitting or walking will probably soon be embarrassing and debilitating. Even coughing or coughing may cause greater pain.

Keeping your anxiety under control

Now you could have a significant role in your pain management by simply keeping your physician and the nursing team informed concerning your annoyance. Most of your will probably be quantified and through your hospital stay, you'll soon be asked to rate your pain on the scale with numbers zero through ten. Zero isn't any hassle and is the worst possible pain. This technique is effective for the healthcare team to discover how a pain control treatment is working or in case there's a requirement to create changes.

Who's may assist you to deal with your anxiety?

Now you as well as your health care provider will chat about your pain control before operation, deciding on what's acceptable for you personally. Sometimes doctors provide at a pain pro to work together with you after your operation.

At the very close of your day, even however, you're one which is likely to create the ultimate choice. Your health history and present health state is going to be employed by your physician and the pain pros to supply you the choices for pain control.

The various forms of pain management treatments

Additionally, it is more typical for an individual to be provided with more than 1 kind of pain control therapy. It's dependent on their wants and the sort of operation they'd had. Your physician and the pain specialist will probably create sure they're safe but effective, however, there's some amount of danger for any kind of drug. A number of the most widely used pain control therapies are:

- **intravenous pca (patient-controlled analgesia)**

Pca is a pump that's automatic and allows the individual to jelling safe levels of pain medication. The machine is programmed and can just release a particular amount within a particular period of time.

- **nerve blocks**

A nerve block controls pain in small, remote parts of the human anatomy. This system of pain control might be spread through an epidural catheter for protracted pain control.

- **cosmetic dentistry medications**

Later operation sooner or later, your physician will probably dictate some kind of pain control medication that's taken orally. You need to allow the nursing staff understand once you're having pain and when it's been over the typical four-hour interval, they provide you with precisely the prescribed dose.

Infection direction without drugs

There are tactics to attain pain control too. Such as directed imagery, a concentrated comfort method is effective by the individual' creating composed and tranquil pictures within their own mind. This emotional escape can also be enriched by hearing music and changing rankings.

Your physician might provide you guidelines for heat and cold therapy. This will diminish your pain and also some other swelling you might well be experiencing. For operation in the chest or abdominal area, employing a pillow for those who personally a cough, sneeze or simply take deep breaths can help being a process of pain control.

One of the best medical problems we frequently face in our day to day life is annoyance. As stated by estimation one-third individuals of earth are confronting issues of pain. Anxiety in just about any one of its kind vastly affects our own life quality. Pain management could be the name of a interdisciplinary approach which re-lives or helps in alleviating pain.

Infection management has distinct methods determined by the kind and potency of pain. In a given pain control team you can find after actors demanded. All these are medical professionals, clinical psychologists, physiotherapists, occupational therapists, nurses and pros etc.

Infection is very painful following a operation notably in orthopedic surgeries pain is sometimes described as an excellent problem for the patient since he could be totally on bed for a few of months. For that reason, pain control is essential for all these patients. Pain management can be necessary like an individual or patient afflicted the pain for quite a while will probably soon be a simple prey for melancholy which is likely to cause his life harder.

Infection is undesirable in its own kind and ought to be suitably handled for easy livings. There are lots of methods available that may assist in tackling the pain. This we shall mostly take in to consideration the pain control methods after a operation.

A pain management strategy after a operation can be multi disciplinary plus it may possibly be united with the input of healthcare professionals, acupuncturists, physiotherapists, chiropractors, clinical therapists and psychologists.

Most pain management methods after operation are dedicated to shared strategies and methods. Listed here are a few methods that actually help control pain after operations are after. Comfort is exceptionally useful feature in pain control and this system patient has been introduced to a relaxed and friendly atmosphere due to their physical and psychological comfort.

Deep breathing, progressive muscular relaxation (PMR) and fanciful gaudiness is useful for comfort. Exercises can also be also utilized to deal with pain after operation. These exercises are extremely simple bodily pursuits. Cold and heat treatments and stress direction can be utilized in several pain control systems.

Infection management may also involve any type of

narcotics. If pain after operation is immense simply than narcotics might be prescribed as narcotics take some side effects together with them which often leads the patient at a challenge if practiced at a standard routine.

Therapies may play vital part in pm (pain control) after operation. Massage can be of assistance to relax the muscle throughout the area of operation plus it'll lower the odds of redness and swelling in operation location. Emotional pain control methods may be practiced to take care of pain after operation. In this respect a proficient psychologist can also be hired which will coordinate together with patient and certainly will bring realistic consequences helping throughout the pm.

Food can be vital in discharging pain. For effective pm after operation an individual need to need to take care concerning the intakes of the patient because they matter. Some hypersensitive attack could occur with a few patients when their food isn't given precisely according to exactly what prescribed by a health care provider.

In case the pain is recurrence following the operation in relation to morphine may be supplied to the individual patient. Morphine is an important chemical in opium that's extremely effective against pain alleviation. It acts on the central nervous system of this patient also can be most widely used medicine for host pain after having a surgical operation. Morphine may be utilized to decrease pain such as chronic pain such as cancer. Tens machines may be employed for pm after having a operation. These machines also give a temporary pain relief in most people but those machines should really be just used with utmost caution.

Pairing chronic pain and storing it under control can be difficult. Most patients aren't certain about the total procedure and way of pain control, which explains the reason why they usually rely upon painkillers and medications for fast relief. In this informative article, we'll discuss pain control and matters which matter the most.

The basics

Chronic pain could be related to numerous illnesses, not limited by gout, unsuspected accidents, cancer treatment, and several other old and unhealed harms. When you've got persistent pain in another of one's own body parts for at least a month which does not appear to improve, you need to think about seeing a pain management physician. There are certainly a large selection of alternatives available, and typically, doctors often rely upon multiple treatments, based on the truth of this situation.

Recognizing pain better

Infection is real, and it may impact various individuals in an alternative way. To get example, when a certain patient is miserable about chronic pain, then his sense and emotional condition will probably differ from somebody else, who's suffered an unexpected harm. The entire process of pain control relies on several criteria. First things first, the doctor will think about the possible requirement for additional evaluation and identification. That can be essential for determining the entire nature and degree of treatment. He may also propose a couple of first items and lifestyle changes, in order to know the answer of this individual. When the pain is overly intense, he might also offer you extra drugs to reduce the inflammation, whilst to lower the total disquiet.

YOGA FOR PAIN RELIEF

Yoga Back Pain, Neck Pain, Shoulder Pain. Finally Find
Relief From Your Acute Or Chronic Pain

William M Wittman

Quotes

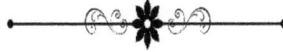

"It's not about being good at something. It's about being good to yourself."

"A flower does not think of competing to the flower next to it. It just blooms."

"Yoga is the journey of the self, through the self, to the self." -- **The Bhagavad Gita**

"You cannot always control what goes on outside. But you can always control what goes on inside."

"The longest journey of any person is the journey inward."

"Yoga is the study of balance, and balance is the aim of all living creatures: it is our home." — Rolf Gates

"Our own physical body possesses a wisdom which we who inhabit the body lack. We give it orders which make no sense."—**Henry Miller**

"Yoga, an ancient but perfect science, deals with the evolution of humanity. This evolution includes all aspects of one's being, from bodily health to self-realization. Yoga means union—the union of body with consciousness and consciousness with the soul. Yoga cultivates the ways of maintaining a balanced attitude in day-to-day life and endows skill in the performance of one's actions." —**B.K.S. Iyengar**

"Do not kill the instinct of the body for the glory of the pose."—**Vanda Scaravelli**

"The body benefits most when the postures are performed consciously and with full understanding. It takes time to accomplish difficult postures. Avoid forcing the body into them prematurely. Work into them gradually. Otherwise, the body can be harmed."—**Swami Kripalu**

"Once your foundation is improved, it is much easier to put the rest of your house in order."—**Leslie Kaminoff,**

"Yoga aims to remove the root cause of all diseases, not to treat its symptoms as medical science generally attempts to do."—**Swami Vishnu-devananda**

"To keep the body in good health is a duty ... otherwise, we shall not be able to keep our mind strong and clear."—**Buddha**

"The breath is the key to unlocking your body's potential."—**Baron Baptiste**

"The secret of health for both mind and body is not to mourn for the past, not to worry about the future, or not to anticipate troubles, but to live in the pose moment wisely and earnestly." — **Buddha**

"Even after you have rolled up your mat, yoga continues"—**ZubinAtre**

INTRODUCTION

This book is a guide to finish the Physical, psychological, and psychological suffering of chronic pain. It's founded on the newest improvements in mind-body research along with also the knowledge of the yoga tradition. This book will provide you a fresh direction of considering the triggers of your own suffering and sensible strategies for stopping your disrelaxation. You are going to find out how your previous experiences with trauma, sickness, and other stressful life events have shifted the way that your head and bodywork together. You'll also understand how these modifications produce chronic physical and psychological pain.

Employing yoga's arsenal of mind-body healing Practices such as breathing, relaxation, movement, and meditation, you'll have the ability to modify your experience of annoyance. As you incorporate yoga into your daily life, your entire body and the brain will turn into a relaxational place to be.

This book is for Anybody experiencing recurrent or chronic pain. Yoga has shown beneficial for all kinds of pain, such as back pain, headache, fibromyalgia, rheumatoid arthritis, and chronic fatigue syndrome, and carpal tunnel syndrome, and irritable bowel syndrome, and premenstrual symptoms, to mention only a couple.

You might not believe your pain will be the worst pain on the planet. Perhaps you've heard to live with this. However, if bodily pain is a relaxational presence on your lifetime, this novel is right for you. This can allow you to alleviate whatever pain you've got and provide you back your power and excitement for life.

Or maybe you believe, "My pain is that the most powerful on the planet, and yoga is not for individuals with pain such as this." However, take heart: Yoga might be the sole factor for pain similar to this. If you are living with severe chronic pain which medication has been not able to take care of, you know you've got the power to endure it. Yoga might not heal the pain, but it is going to allow you to perform more than endure it. Yoga can help you recover your life by providing back a feeling of relaxation and control within your body and mind, whether the pain goes away.

This book can be for anybody who would like to know or assist somebody with chronic pain. In case you've got a loved one with chronic pain, then you may use the thoughts and techniques in this book to encourage her or him. Yoga instructors, physical therapists, therapists, and other health care professionals may add a varied set of resources to their curative toolbox. Every chapter shares not only strategies and solutions but actual insight to the essence of chronic pain. The stories from this book will Provide you an appreciation for what it's like to undergo chronic pain and also thoughts to the yoga can be adapted to meet particular needs of people.

Though this book Targets chronic physical distress, pain comprises not only body aches but additionally heartaches. Since you will know, both of these varieties of pain aren't completely unrelated encounters. Both contemporary science, along with the yoga tradition teach us there is not any clear dividing line between bodily pain, for example, chronic low back pain, along with psychological pain, like depression. Both kinds of pain have been from the brain and the human body, and the two kinds of pain react to some mind-body approach such as yoga. You'll come to realize the ideas and practices within this book may also help you cope with anger, nervousness, depression, and depression.

There are a couple of things more annoying to a individual who has chronic pain than hearing someone say,"Your pain is in your head" How frequently have you heard anything similar to that and wanted that the individual stating it might dwell in your own body for only 1 day feel exactly what you believe, and also know-how actual your annoyance is?

But what if those words were really the secret to Relieving your distress?

Persistent pain is on mind, but this doesn't imply That which you think it means. The experience of pain is real. Your pain gets a biological foundation. It is only that the origin of your pain is not confined to where you are feeling or in which you think it's coming out of. It is not only on your shoulder, your spine, or your buttocks. It is not only a issue with your muscles or joints.

For years, scientists and physicians believed that pain may be caused exclusively by harm to the construction of their human body. They looked for its origin of chronic pain at thoracic spinal disks, muscular injuries, and illnesses. More recent research, but points to another supply of chronic pain: that the exact actual biology of your ideas, feelings, expectations, along with even memories. A lot of chronic pain has its own origins in a concrete injury or sickness, but it's sustained by the way that first injury affects, not only the human body but also the mind-body connection.

We typically think of their brain as somehow Separate from your system. The brain is that this mysterious encounter we have of becoming : it is what we believe, how we sense, and also our capacity to act with conscious aim. But here is what: your brain is on your physique. Sensations, feelings, ideas they take place within the entire body. Each feeling notion and the choice is its very own biochemical function within the entire body, delivering hormones, and activity signals travelling across the body.

Sensations, ideas, and feelings are generated and conveyed by several Systems of the human body, including the nervous system, the endocrine system, and also the immune system. Every one these approaches are closely connected to one another. Together, they write the biological mind. Their interactions make your own expertise of sensation, ideas, and feelings, including bodily pain and the way they work together, are also the secret to end your pain.

Finding out that an issue is more complicated. Than you initially thought doesn't normally come as a nice surprise. However, the sophistication of chronic pain is really excellent news.

This means that attempting To resolve the entire body with operations, pain drugs, or physical treatment isn't your only hope. If you're like most other individuals with chronic pain, all these rigorously body-based strategies have aided just minimally or neglected. Whenever your body pain can be connected to what's happening in your thoughts, attempting to resolve the entire body without damaging your mind won't ever provide you full aid.

For a Lot of People, the biggest shock of all is you don't even have to understand exactly what, if anything, is wrong with the human physique. If the doctors can not let you know exactly what is causing your pain, then you do not have to wait a diagnosis to begin recovery. Awareness of the way that your head and bodywork collectively will provide you a much more potent comprehension of your annoyance compared to any identification you'll be able to get. With this new knowledge, the practice of recovery can start quickly, having something as straightforward as a breathing meditation or exercise.

Why Yoga

The energy of Yoga lies in the convention's profound Comprehension of the mind-body relationship. possibly promoted in books as a means to supply you with a fantastic body, but the goal of conventional is to reestablish the health of body and serenity of mind.

While is now Famous for its hard bodily postures, such as the headstand or even the lotus posethat you won't observe any of these advanced postures within this book. They've got little to do with alleviating chronic pain.

Instead, you can Learn a broad selection of techniques which reflect the complete reach of its therapeutic tools. Before long you'll find that if you can breathe, you can do . If it's possible to focus on your ideas and feelings, then you are able to do . If you're inclined to explore the body feels and the way to look after it, then it is possible to do .isn't about turning your body in unrelaxationable postures; also you're able to exercise even in the event that you can't get out of bed.

These simple practices Will direct you on the route of finishing your suffering. will teach you how you can concentrate your mind to modify your experience of bodily pain. It may teach you how you can change feelings of despair, frustration, stress, and anger. It may teach you how you can obey your body and look after your requirements so you can take part in the actions that matter for you. It may provide you back the feeling of security, management, and courage which you want to proceed beyond the own experience of chronic pain.

Within this book. We are going to start by researching A mind-body perspective of pain which has its origins at the practice, however, is encouraged by an increasing body of research from neuroscience, psychology, and medicine.

The fundamental assumption of This book is that a lot of our regular, chronic disrelaxation is a heard mind-body reaction. Stress begins with one occasion, but it's sustained by how accidents, diseases, and other traumatic incidents alter the body and mind. The body and mind do not only recover from these types of events--they understand from them. The body and mind normally conform to previous risks by getting overprotective. An accident to the trunk may cause the chronic hypersensitivity of a spinal nerve. Traumatic life experience affects how in which the brain processes strain and stress. In the long run, these adaptations"warn" you about dangers that no longer exist and also direct one to overreact to new adventures. This procedure keeps you into a condition of chronic pain, nervousness, or prevention.

The tradition Recognized this practice of mind-body learning before modern science can quantify it from the nervous system. In , customs learned from previous experiences are known as samskaras. doctrine teaches that sanskaras are in the origin of unnecessary distress, and exercise is the very best method to unlearn them.

This book is dedicated to instructing you techniques which can help you unlearn customs of distress and make new recovery habits of body and mind. emphasizes the inherent capacity every individual must undergo joy and health. practices are the resources to wake up this capability and cure your pain.

We Start with this breathtaking , that's the fundamental instrument of recovery in the tradition. You are going to find out to use simple breath awareness to develop a feeling of control and security at any time, for example, intense pain. You will learn feel-good moves that enhance the ease and quality of your breathing in regular life, and you're going to discover specific breathing methods for handling pain.

The following step to Recovery is befriending the human own body . You are going to find out to obey your own body and develop awareness on what it requires. Meditation practices for creating peace with your own body can allow you to conquer the anger, despair, and frustration, which are typical answers to chronic pain.

Befriending your own body and researching the breath can prepare one for studying the bodily exercises of proceeding with the breath (vinyasa) and carrying moves and poses (asana). You will discover a fundamental sequence of motions which were demonstrated to help decrease pain and restore bodily health and operate. You will also know how to make a private movement practice that satisfies your requirements and is safe on the human entire body.

Next, you'll find out how to experience deep relaxation , that can be essential to unlearning chronic muscle strain, stress sensitivity, stress, and stress. Last, you will learn a few meditation methods, each targeting a particular facet of chronic pain, in handling pain feeling to changing hard feelings. Both meditation and relaxation can allow you to tap in the human body's natural healing responses along with the brain's innate ability to experience happiness.

When You've had a Opportunity to test 's therapeutic techniques, we will have a look at how to make part of your daily life. In the previous chapter of the book, you will find out how to create into a protective Yoga practice which develops the awareness of relaxation, strength, guts, and energy, a"first aid" healing practice for when you're in physical or psychological pain, and techniques for incorporating your favourite healing methods of into everyday life.

CHAPTER ONE

❧

WHAT IS PAIN

Three major ideas in the past couple of Decades of pain study have hugely improved our comprehension of chronic pain. First came the realization that pain is really a mind-body procedure, formed not only by bodily illness and injury but also by ideas, feelings, stress, and studying. The 2nd key understanding was that if pain becomes persistent, it plays with the very same principles as a standard healthier pain reaction. The concluding progress was the expanding understanding of the way to get the brain and body's organic pain-suppressing methods via breathing, meditation, relaxation, or motion.

These three thoughts --today Commonly accepted in the health care area --help explain the reason why pain becomes constant and everything you could do on it. Even though the contemporary mind-body perspective of chronic pain is more complicated, its complexity makes it loaded with opportunities for recovery. Since you read about the numerous elements that form the experience of pain, then you are able to have a look at everyone as a route for altering up your experience of annoyance.

Before We investigate why and how the pain system goes awry in chronic pain, and let us look for a second how beneficial the pain process is if it works.

Despite its poor Standing, pain is an elegant illustration of the mind-body relationship. A world with no pain could be a risky location. Pain tells you whenever your physical security and well-being are in danger. It compels one to guard yourself when you're being hurt. And it makes it possible to learn how to prevent things that may hurt you.

How can pain do these things? It coordinates a Mind-body reaction that sends your focus and energy into the most significant job at hand: shielding your self.

The protective pain Response starts when the body undergoes some physical danger, like a cut, burn, or even swollen muscle. This threat is detected by technical nerves in skin, joints, tendons, and organs which listen for signals that your system is at risk. When all is secure on the planet, these hazard sensors are silent. However, when there's harm or injury, they deliver a hazard sign during the spinal cord and up into the mind.

When danger Signs arrive in the field of your mind that receives sensory information, so the mind does a sort of evaluation. What is happening? How severe is that? Is this something I want to look closely at? In case the mind makes the decision to look closely at this incoming signals, the message gets delivered to many different regions of the mind which is able to enable you to respond to a crisis. This system of brain regions has been known as the"painneuromatrix" (Melzack 2001); however, you can imagine this like a public address system. The data travels out to nearly anybody who may need it or understand exactly what to do for this.

Including the Areas of the brain that change the danger signals into pain senses, and that means you understand just what is occurring within the body. The message also has sent into the regions of your mind that keep an eye on battle and goals. This focuses your attention on what's wrong and makes you problem-solving of what you could do to make things easier. Emotion-processing regions of the brain also receive the concept, triggering a vast assortment of responses, from fear of anger. These feelings, but not agreeable, play an significant part in motivating one to guard yourself. Combined, your ideas and feelings concerning the bodily senses of pain compose the enduring part of the complete pain encounter. This sense that something's wrong is your mind's strategy for ensuring you do whatever that you can to keep your self protected.

As a result of the pain reaction, you are Feeling pretty gloomy and encouraged to do something to end the pain and disrelaxation. That is where stress comes from. To assist you do it, the danger signals happen to be concurrently routed into the regions of the brain that assist the body establish a crisis pressure reaction.

The emergency pressure Response coordinates the activities of their nervous system, endocrine system, and immune system--that which a few investigators have predicted a"supersystem of stress" (Chapman, Tuckett, along with Woo Song 2008). This supersystem participates in to save the day (or, at the least your lifetime) by activating a cascade of physiological adjustments that provide you the power and attention to guard yourself from life-threatening danger. The nervous system raises your sympathetic stimulation, frees up your pulse and blood pressure, heightening your senses, raising muscle strain, and flood your system with energy in the shape of fats and sugars in your blood. The endocrine system releases adrenaline and other stress hormones into the blood, which further heightens the effects of the sympathetic nervous system. The immune system becomes prepared to heal any wounds or combat any poisonous invaders by boosting inflammation through the body and triggering immune cells that protect against disease. These modifications might leave you feeling stressed, on edge, and also exposed, but they also prepare the body for fast thinking and activity, which can be very beneficial in a crisis.

Even following the danger Is gone, the pain reaction isn't over. The body and mind are extremely interested in ensuring you are aware of how to safeguard yourself from the danger later on. Thus the nervous system starts the practice of learning from that adventure.

If the pain has been important, this usually entails A psychological replay of this event long after it's over-- remembering that the pain, telling folks about the annoyance, examining exactly what occurred, and considering what you can do in order to steer clear of similar pain later on. It can be tough to quit considering the pain or stressing about if it is going to return or get worse.

Most Men and Women think of That rumination as being different from the pain reaction, but it's an significant part the protective procedure. Stress's imprint in your Ideas and memory aids you learn in the pain experience, which makes it more Probable that You'll Be motivated and able to avoid a similar hazard from the future. Obviously, while you're Seeing the interrelated ideas, it does not feel so beneficial.

But understanding these ideas are so difficult to shake might allow you to be hard on yourself if they develop. Knowing that your brain is turning stories to keep you secure also can make you less inclined to trust that the worst-case situation your head paints.

The nervous system is. Additionally performing its learning process out your conscious awareness. Any sort of illness or injury, even one that's short-lived or seems to be completely cured, can alter how the nervous system processes pain. The body doesn't only heal an illness or injury; however, learns from it also uses the expertise to forecast the future. Each part of the nervous system, out of hazard sensors in the human anatomy to nerves in the mind, will accommodate in ways Which Make It easier to discover a similar danger from the long run and bracket a protective pain reaction

It's this Complete set of protective mind reactions --from the very first pain sensations To difficulty, psychological suffering, stress reaction, and learningthat generates your private experience of annoyance. Much more than only a physical feeling, pain is just one of the very complexes of individual experiences. That is the reason why pain reaches into each element of your own life, affecting the way you feel, think, and behave.

Overall, the Protective pain reaction isn't a terrible system for success in severe emergencies And managing short-term pain. Regrettably, the things Which Make pain so Powerful At helping us live in a dangerous universe would be the very things which produce chronic Pain so intricate and thus persistent. Let us consider now what happens When the protective pain reaction turns into chronic pain and what you could do on it.

ACUTE PAIN VERSUS CHRONIC PAIN

Among the very first things to understand about chronic pain is the fact that it doesn't stick to the principles of this normal acute pain reaction described previously. Knowing the distinction between acute pain and chronic pain would be crucial to your capacity to reduce and handle your pain.

Intense pain is a direct and temporary Reaction To some sort of illness or injury. As explained above, it starts with a true danger to the human body and contributes to a fair protective reaction. Intense pain isalso, for the large part, a fairly reliable indicator of this danger for your entire body. Should you bump your leg, then you may feel immediate pain in which you're hurt. If you set your hands on a hot stove, then you may feel pain wherever your skin fulfils harmful heat. Generally, the power of the pain will probably suit the seriousness of this danger --the worse the danger, the worse the own pain. After the danger is finished and the entire body is treated, the pain goes off. In summary: if you are feeling severe pain, then you can presume there is a fantastic link between what you're feeling and what's happening to the human body.

Many people, including many men and women that you might have spoke to about your own pain, consider this can be how chronic pain functions. The premise is when you've got chronic pain; then you need a chronic danger within the body which has been alert your mind. And when your pain gets worse, then it has to be since the danger from the body is becoming worse.

With Chronic pain, which is seldom the situation. Persistent pain differs from acute pain in several significant ways. To begin with, the body is able to be sensitive to danger, sending risk signals to the mind even if the danger is slight or nonexistent. Secondly, the mind can become prone to translate situations as threatening and senses as debilitating, making pain reactions which are out of proportion to any actual threat. Ultimately, with recurrent pain encounters, the bounds between many characteristics of the pain reaction --feeling, distress, and stress--becoming blurred. This permits any of these to activate a full-size protective pain reaction.

These differences imply That chronic pain is a much less reliable sign about what is occurring in your own body than severe pain. The pain you are feeling can reflect a legitimate threat to your system, but only as frequently, it doesn't. What It does signify is that a protective mind-body reaction. That's become overprotective. In most cases of chronic pain, both the body and mind have Learned well the way to discover the slightest sign of a hazard and bracket a Complete protective reaction in all of its glory of suffering and pain.

Chronic pain does not Simply make you more sensitive to bodily pain--it may make you sensitive to any sort of bodily, psychological, or social stress. This greater sensitivity can be thanks to neuroplasticity. Every pain experience, which triggers a stress reaction strengthens the stress reaction. Repeated pain encounter leads to greater sensitivity of those regions of the mind which detect not just pain senses but all sorts of conflict and danger. This sort of learning can play a massive part in the way chronic physical pain may develop into chronic psychological distress, such as stress disorders and depression.

Does chronic stress makes you more vulnerable to chronic stress; however, chronic stress will make you sensitive to bodily pain. The bodily changes of this stress reaction (like inflammation and stimulation) provide the ideal learning environment for your body and mind, raising the odds that the pain will end up persistent. Persistent stress can, consequently, lead to precisely the exact modifications to the nervous system as bodily pain experience: hazard sensors from the human body become more sensitive, and the nervous system much more excited to manoeuvre those risk signals into the brain, and the mind more inclined to interpret senses as debilitating.

When It's becoming hard for You to Keep pain and Stress different in your head, imagine what: the nervous system has the exact same trouble. As pain and stress are survival methods, and since they often go together, the nervous system is able to begin to take care of all risks --physical, psychological, financial, societal, etc. --such as physical pain.

Each time you have a Pain reaction, your mind is constructing connections between the several unique senses, ideas, feelings, and also cues on your surroundings that come together with the experience of annoyance. Whenever these connections are powerful, whatever your mind associates with bodily pain--stress, anger, and lack of sleep, and the memory of stress, anxieties about the long term, etc. --may trigger a whole protective pain reaction: senses, distress, and all of. A pain reaction may also be triggered by risks that haven't anything to do with previous pain along with your entire body, like stress on the job or even a fight with a relative. Even more astonishingly, emotional dangers can cause pain-inducing adjustments to your system. By way of instance, stress was proven to activate a exceptional pattern of muscular strain in people with chronic lower back pain (Glombiewski, Tersek, along with Rief 2008). In spite of the normal pain reaction, chronic physical pain can begin in the mind and operate its way into the remainder of the human body.

The Most Crucial take-home point from All This study is that stressIs a huge portion of chronic pain. It's both a result and cause of headache and also --for many people--a chronic state of its very own. Because of this, learning the way to decrease stress is going to be among the most crucial actions that you take in treating and dealing with chronic pain. A number of the things which reduce stress, like a feeling of control, social assistance, and meditation, and could also decrease physical strain. Focusing on those items can be more effective for chronic pain than attempting to determine what's wrong with your own human body and the way to repair it.

Regardless of what seems like a hefty dose of terrible information about chronic pain, you will find just two really major reasons to be optimistic.

The first is the Body and mind have built-in therapeutic responses which are equally as strong as their protective pain-and-stress answers. These curing responses comprise the human body's natural pain-suppressing techniques, the relaxation response, along with positive feelings such as happiness and gratitude. You are able to learn how to trigger these answers to offset the consequences of stress and pain and also help your system recover from illness and injury.

The next rationale for Trust is that learning is life-threatening, and not one of the modifications you have learned need to become permanent. Sensitivity to stress and pain can eventually become resilience. Neuroplasticity may be exploited for recovery. Your body and mind have discovered how to"perform" chronic pain, and your task is to teach it something fresh.

Both of these motives for Expect are what the remainder of this novel is all about. You Have a better comprehension of the factors contributing to chronic pain; however, the most crucial advice is to come. You may Find out more about all them Healing answers in the chapters which follow, With clear advice about the best way best to use these to decrease your disrelaxation and cure Your own pain.

REUNITING THE MIND, BODY, AND SPIRIT

While neuroscience, psychology, and Medication are becoming better at describing why and the pain stays, they don't yet have pleasing answers. Stress drugs fail within the long run more frequently than not. Stress management programs often concentrate on dealing with pain instead of altering the pain encounter.

This is where yoga comes in. The yoga tradition has evolved as a method to stop unnecessary suffering. This guarantee was explained as far back as two thousand decades back from the Yoga Sutras, among the earliest guides to this goal and practice of yoga.

Yoga Philosophy provides hope for freedom from suffering, and also its own practices supply the resources for recovery. This chapter will introduce you to a number of the crucial ideas in the yoga tradition, which will direct you in your way to end unnecessary pain and disrelaxation. These notions breathe soul into the science explained in chapter 1 and extend a frame for comprehending the practices you are going to learn from the chapters which follow.

Contemporary science has shown that That which we call"the brain" isn't separate from that which we call"the entire body " This is a great basis for a holistic outlook; however, it leaves something crucial about exactly what it has to be person: soul.

Yoga Adds this missing facet. As stated by the yoga practice, the body isn't simply mind and body but can also be breath, intellect, and happiness. Breath is the life force which amuses you; intellect is the internal manual; delight is your link to something larger than yourself. Collectively, these 3 measurements capture the concept of soul. In addition, they point to what's so often lacking from a normal scientific or medical standpoint: every individual's inherent capacity of recovery and well-being.

This yogic version of mind, body, and soul was described Tens of thousands of years back, but its perspectives are equally important now. As the scientific version recognizes that mind and body Can't be split, the yogic version acknowledges

This body, Mindsoul are connected as a single whole. All five measurements mind, body, breath, intellect, and pleasure are equally significant in understanding a individual's health. Imbalances in any of those measurements can affect others, and healing occurring in anyone may disperse to others.

Breath

From the conventional Language of yoga, the word for breath and life force is exactly the same: prana. Prana is the power which supports all you do, belief, and texture. It comes in the breath, however, is revived by the entire body.

Yogis Consider the flow of prana within your own body is the thing that enables your body to cure. If prana is reduced, you can feel exhausted, ill, miserable, or in distress. If prana is large, you are feeling more lively, joyful, and powerful. The circulation of prana within your body may be affected by whatever which you put into your own body --drink, food, drugs --and anything which you do with the human entire body, such as exercise, sleep, and function. On the other hand, the very best connection to prana is that the very simple act of breathing. Bearing this in mind, it's simple to learn how the level of your breathing may affect your well-being.

Since the breath is The basis for prana, the yoga tradition has generated many breathing methods to encourage the entire life force, which flows through you. These breathing techniques are known as pranayama, which actually translates to"energyadministration " This is a great way to consider the breathing techniques that you are going to learn in this book. They're tools for encouraging your vitality, mood, and well-being.

The breath--since it Supports prana--is fundamental to each yoga practice you are going to learn from the book. This is why we'll begin your yoga course together with breath knowledge and pranayama practices within another phase.

Wisdom

The Majority of us are Utilized to Looking out of ourselves for advice. We turn to specialists, police, physicians, and also yes, even writers. That is fine once you will need to collect specialized advice or remarks. However, the yoga tradition maintains that there's an internal guide that exceeds the collective wisdom of specialists. This internal wisdom will tell you about what's true for you, and the way you are able to experience peace of mind, more than any external authority may ever understand.

From the yogic version of the body, mind, and soul, Intellect is more about instinct

And mindfulness compared to about understanding Or intellect. It's the capability to check out what's authentic in this period and what's required in this instant. It's also the capability to determine through the customs of the brain -- such as stress, failure, self- criticism, and also stress --which create distress. Yoga teaches that each individual has this capacity and it's an significant part who you're

You can acquire this capacity by paying more attention to the internal advice of your breath, body, ideas, and feelings. Meditation, and meditation particularly, will instruct you how you can differentiate between advice from internal wisdom and favourable habits of their mind. Exercising also grows your self-care instinct, so assisting you to know what your body should be healthy and without the pain. If you reconnect with this advice, you'll have a profound source of insight and strength for dealing with life's troubles.

Joy

Yoga Identifies pleasure --a pure awareness of well-being, gratitude, and peace--because the strangest aspect of what it means to be human. You may have felt this type of pleasure at particular moments in your own life --the arrival of your child, the opinion of a pond, or even while rapping in creative or hands-on work. These glimpses aren't determined by outside events. It's just better to be in contact with your normal condition of well-being in such specific moments.

From the yogic perspective, delight is the nearest to what you could Call your authentic character. It's not a fast-changing, fast-disappearing joy that changes according to your own ideas, disposition, and current conditions. By comparison, the capacity to feel peace in this instant is fundamental to who you really are. This internal joy is not as vulnerable to the fluctuations in your own life, and it isn't determined by fixing what's incorrect or becoming what you would like. Even chronic pain can't eliminate your capacity to sense this section of your self.

Yoga practice makes it possible to reconnect with the inner pleasure. When It's a meditation On gratitude, a relaxation pose which places the human body and head at ease, Or a breathing exercise which reinforces the flow of energy into your Human anatomy --they share the advantage of bringing You back into a normal awareness of well-being.

SUFFERING AND TRANSFORMATION (SAMSKARA)

If joy and wisdom are as much part of You as your body and breath, why would it be so easy to become disconnected from those organic conditions? Both contemporary yoga and science discuss precisely the identical response to this issue: current pain and disrelaxation has its origins previously pain, injury, stress, reduction, and sickness.

Persistent pain and Suffering tend to be learned answers based on previous experiences. Contemporary science uses words such as neuroplasticity to spell out the procedure for learning from previous experiences; yoga utilizes the phrase samskara. Samskaras are the memories of their human body and brain that affect the way individuals experience the pose time. Yoga doctrine teaches that each and every encounter you've --such as your own ideas, feelings, and senses --leaves a hint to the human body, mind, and soul. Each encounter is saved as a lesson learned about lifestyle.

These classes Aren't Only a listing of everything you've undergone; they are, in addition, a blueprint for how you are going to respond to new adventures. Samskaras been the customs of their human body and thoughts that make you more inclined to replicate your previous experiences and activities and more inclined to translate the world through the filter of your own previous experiences. These customs help keep you stuck, feeling the very same emotions, thinking the very same thoughts, as well as experiencing the identical pain.

Yoga is a process of positive transformation

Samskaras don't Always cause distress; they can also cause positive change. Just as injury, sickness, pain, and stress leave traces on your own human body and head, so do positive encounters. Relaxation, relaxation, joyous motion, gratitude, along with other positive ideas and emotions, alter your entire body, mind, and soul. Everything you exercise, you encounter. Everything you exercise, you're.

From the Yoga Sutras, the yogic sage PatanjaliProvides the following guidance about the best way best to alter samskaras:"Should you would like to be with some negative habit of the head, blatantly practice its reverse" (vitarkabadhanepratipakshabhavanam). To put it differently, if you'd like to be free of distress due to old habits, then you want to practice something fresh.

Yoga is really a time-tested method for changing your habits of mind and body. Yoga training interrupts the samskaras that result in distress and helps them with positive new habits of mind and body. Yoga's method of changing samskaras is easy and straightforward: you, practice consciousness of the habit and the way that it contributes to distress, and 2, practice its reverse and detect if that reduces your distress.

To Simply take a very simple example, imagine you wanted to become free of this pain brought on by a learned habit of holding tension on your neck. Yoga would allow you to do just two Items: first, to become mindful of if And in which you hold tension within the entire body, including the neck, and also the way the tension contributes to distress; and secondly, to find out to breathe and extend to relax your neck and give up the strain which makes you more inclined to hold stress in your entire body.

This Procedure Is the foundation for each and every practice within this book. Each yoga exercise is a chance to make a brand new, positive hint on the human body, mind, and soul. You'll be guided on how best to recognize the habits of mind and body that lead to chronic pain and disrelaxation.

You'll be guided in the way to give up every habit and actively exercise its therapeutic reverse via breathing, motion, relaxation, or meditation.

The Tools of Transformation

The yoga tradition includes Lots of tools for conversion, and also the very best method to find that will work great for you will be to research all them.

In this book, you may be introduced into a vast selection of standard yoga techniques adapted to your distinctive difficulties of chronic pain. Collectively, these practices tackle each part of mind, body, and soul and can assist you in a condition of wellness, wholeness, and enjoyment.

Let your instinct guide you as you research the practices in every single chapter. Once you discover a practice that cares for you personally, stick with it for a short time. Repeat it each single day. Watch how it affects your experience of the physique. Watch how it affects your ideas and feelings. See whether it leads to additional changes in your lifetime.

Yoga Teaches the five dimensions of human experience-- breath, body, thoughts, intellect, and pleasure --are profoundly interconnected. To stop suffering, you can begin anywhere and allow the recovery work its way through each layer of your mind, body, and soul. A yoga exercise that requires the breath because its beginning point will affect every element of the human body. A meditation which takes the brain as its beginning point will provide you access to a internal wisdom and allow you to reconnect with a normal state of pleasure. A motion exercise which takes the human body and breath because its beginning point can grow to be a moving meditation which calms the brain. Any practice within this novel may be the key that unlocks the complete therapeutic benefits of yoga.

You can add other yoga Practices with the years, as you discover an increasing number of techniques which inspire you and help you handle your pain.

SCIENCE OF NECK PAIN

Even though Back pain generally controls more focus --in part, since it contributes to much more work-related handicap --neck pain is almost as common. Consider these figures in the Bone and Joint Decade 2000--2010 Task Force on Neck Pain and Its Associated Disorders (Haldeman, Carroll, and Cassidy 2008)an Global set of practician-scientists found in 2000 within their World Health Organization's international initiative focusing on behavioural disorders:

Most Folks can expect to undergo a certain amount of neck pain within their lifetimes (Haldeman et al.. 2008).

Up to 70 percent of individuals report experiencing neck pain within the last calendar year, as well as 45 percent report experiencing neck pain within the previous month (Hogg-Johnson et al.. 2008).

About 5% of all North Americans report being handicapped due to neckdisrelaxation, and the other 10 percent report undergoing low-level handicap together with long-term neck pain (Lidgren 2008). Back in Europe, studies demonstrate that chronic or persistent neck pain affects 10 to 20% of their people (ibid.). Each Year, 11 to 14.1% of employees report being restricted in their

Activities due to neck pain (Côté et al.., 2008). Neck pain

is common in most occupational classes, and worker's compensation information seems to considerably underestimate the weight Of neck pain in employees (ibid.) .

Most Individuals with neck pain don't encounter a comprehensive resolution of symptoms (Haldeman et al.. 2008). Between 50 and 85% of these originally undergoing neck pain may report neck pain one to five decades after (ibid.) .

Neck pain and its own Associated ailments --such as aggravation and pain radiating into the top trunk and torso -- are a great deal more prevalent than anyone previously thought, according to the Task Force report, which had been printed in a special supplement to Spine diary (Lidgren 2008). Really, neck-related pain has come to be a significant source of disability across the planet, according to the experts, who noticed that the issue wasn't well known and has been, oftentimes, rather hard to control.

RISK FACTORS FOR NECK PAIN

After undertaking a comprehensive inspection Of the scientific literature about neck pain, in addition to conducting several initial research jobs, the Task Force concluded that neck pain includes a"multifactorialaetiology" (Hogg-Johnson et al.. 2008); or in layman's terms, a number of risk factors may lead to the issue. Some elements which put you at risk for neck pain are out of the control, for example, next (ibid.) :

Age:The Danger for neck pain grows with age up to a summit in midlife (forty to fifty-four) then declines in after decades.

Gender: The Relationship between sex and neck pain seems to change based on the sort of neck disrelaxation. Studies indicate that men are somewhat more inclined to look at a hospital to get a neck sprain or trauma, frequently associated with a traumatic event such as getting hurt when playing sports or performing physical labour. By comparison, girls showed greater levels of visits to your healthcare centre for neckpain, that has been not as inclined to be associated with one particular, problematic event.

Genetics: genetics Heredity Seems to play a role in neck pain, Even Though the mechanics of This connection aren't understood.

Other variables that Affecta individual's risk of neck pain have been controllable, including the following:

Smoking and ecological exposure to cigarette increases the risk of neckdisrelaxation since this can reduce the oxygen content In cells and lead to Emotional issues (ibid.) .

Workplace pressure ,such as high socioeconomic job demands, low social support at work, Sedentary workplace, repetitive work, and accuracy function all raise the chance of neck pain (Côté et al.. 2008).

Physical activity involvement protects against neck pain, because routine Exercisers have a tendency to be fit and springy, and improves the outlook for recovery in neck pain (Hogg-Johnson et al.. 2008).

Astonishingly, the Task Force found no evidence that shared Degenerative changes in the cervical spine are a risk factor for neck pain (ibid.) . The term,"frequent degenerative modifications," describes the slow deterioration of the cartilage that protects the joints, and this happens with age. This condition, called osteoarthritis, frequently referred to as"bronchial arthritis," is actually the most common kind of arthritis. These age-related arthritic fluctuations are a normal fact of life, also from age fifty-five to forty, the majority of us have degenerative changes in the backbone (Haldeman 2008). In most individuals, this can be a benign procedure. But when found on X-ray or MRI, those inevitable modifications are generally labelled degenerative joint disorder , a frightening-sounding identification for something which's normally a benign part of becoming older. If you call a thing a"disorder," it is natural to go trying to find a cure, and also a complete body of literature is different depending on the premise that preventing and persistent neck pain is related to degenerative changes in the cervical spinal column. But because the Task Force found no evidence to confirm that premise, they suggested a new method of studying and tagging neck pain.

Fresh conceptual model of neck pain

Instead,Than see neck pain for a disorder, which regularly sends individuals to a fruitless search for a magical remedy, the Task Force suggested a change in perspective that believes neck pain a happening of life affected by risk factors, a lot of which we could control. According to their extensive analysis, this brand new conceptual design centresaround enabling people to take part in their care.

To Put It Differently, if You are like the great majority of individuals with neck pain, so there are steps that you can take to help safeguard yourself and prevent enabling neck pain interfere with your daily life. By way of instance, the Task

Force discovered that generally speaking, those items which keep you going are great,such as manual and exercise therapy, a umbrella phrase for hands-on physiological therapies like massage, myofascial release, and joint exploitation.

In contrast, normally Those items that block you from moving are poor,such as collars and bed rest. A few other therapies appear valuable, the Task Force noted (Haldeman et al.. 2008), such as instructional movies, low- level laser treatment, and acupuncture. Interventions that focus on recovering work and returning to operate whenever you possibly were usually more powerful than those with no attention.

Top self-care practices comprise Quitting smoking, maintaining Staying active, and keeping favourable thought processes. Research suggests that individuals with poor mental health that are inclined to stress and become frustrated or angry in reaction to neck disrelaxation had a poorer outlook, while people who were optimistic and also had a working style that entailed self-assurance Were prone to undergo pain relief (Côté et al.. 2008). Yoga may be especially beneficial as it keeps you active, alleviates stress, And enhances mood.

Red-Flag Symptoms

While self-care is your best remedy For the great majority of individuals who undergo neck pain, particular"red-flag" signs could be signs of serious conditions--for example cancer, diabetes, fracture, or disease --also signal the need for medical care. It is a Good Idea to consult a physician if you are concerned about your neck pain, andit's vital to seek medical care if you've red-flag symptoms like:

Numbness, tingling, or weakness in your hand or arm

Pain brought on by an accident, injury, or dismiss

Swollen glands Or a lump on your neck

Difficulty breathing or swallowing

Check with your doctor, also, in case you've got a condition that could make you prone to severe neck injury, for example, previous oral hygiene, history of cancer, rheumatoid arthritis, or bone loss due to obesity or corticosteroid therapy.

How Yoga May Assist

Yoga is a deep method of holistic healing which Originated over five million decades back from India. The term"yoga" comes from the ancient Sanskrit term yuj, meaning to"yoke" or"combine," and the practice was made to unify several things. In the most elementary level, yoga aids combine mind and body. In a deeper level, yoga attempts to combine the individual with the generic.

When folks in the West state"yoga," they are commonly Speaking about hatha yoga, 1 branch of the ancient discipline which focuses primarily on bodily postures, breathing exercises, and meditation. Hatha yoga teaches you how you can relax and release stress, in addition, to strengthen weak muscles and extend tight ones. Additionally, it helps to balance and integrate body, mind, and soul so as to boost energy flow and also stimulate the body's own all-natural healing processes.

A Frequent misconception Is that yoga is just for the fit and flexible, and needs one to twist into a pretzel and put in your mind. Among the most common comments, I hear if folks understand I teach yoga would be,"Oh, so I might not do yoga; I am not flexible ," to that I normally respond,"That is like believing your home is too cluttered to employ a maid."

In reality, the sole requirement for practising yoga will be having the capability to breathe!I've Taught yoga for individuals with a vast assortment of health issues, such as cancer, cardiovascular disease, arthritis, arthritis, blindness, fibromyalgia, back pain, congestive heart failure, along with leg amputation. While innovative postures such as headstand are a part of this yoga exercise for a number of individuals, they are by no means needed. Your yoga training ought to be tailored to match your skills and requirements. For a lot of people, yoga entails simple yet strong meditative movements that anybody can do.

Yoga Is Medicine

When most Men and Women Consider medication, they imagine something Material, such as, for instance, a tablet computer to be hauled, an liquid to be consumed, or a shot to be suffered. Some may also think of tests, surgery, or processes to be medication because these high tech manoeuvres will help diagnose and cure illness. Nevertheless, the ancient yogis recognized a fact that contemporary medicine now affirms: easy movement provides deep therapeutic benefits. Now, this belief is adopted by traditional healers and contemporary scientists, both Eastern and Western doctors alike: proper movement enhances wellbeing, whilst firming disturbs it.

To Put It Differently, Motion is medication. And it is a medication that is extremely successful, totally free (or inexpensive), low threat, commercially accessible, socially

Okay, and easy to perform. The primary "side effect" is feeling and looking better. In reality, Dr Robert Butler, founding director of the National Institute on Aging, is fond of stating,"If exercise could be packaged with a pill, it could be one most widely prescribed, and also valuable, medication in the state" (Butler 2009). All it requires to attain significant health benefits is routine exercise.

Within the last few decades, Western Medication Has recognized the healing power of motion and prescribed physical action as a safe and efficient remedy to help prevent, alleviate, and at times even cure a plethora of ailments. Strong scientific proof (U.S. Department of Health and Human Services 2008) files exercise therapeutic advantages in decreasing the chance of, or assisting cure, over two dozen ailments, such as coronary disease, diabetes, and certain cancers (colon, breast, pancreaticcancer, and prostate cancer), hypertension, and arthritis, and depression, obesity, higher cholesterol, stroke, and asthma, and sleep apnea, obesity, and sexual dysfunction.

Physical action, in the Shape of postures And breathing techniques, is a fundamental part of yoga; however, the practice is a great deal more than only a workout. Yoga is a potent type of mind-body medication that approaches wellbeing in a holistic fashion, recognizing that bodily disorders have psychological and spiritual elements. By way of instance, neck pain can involve a vast selection of contributing factors which range from poor posture, weak muscles, and persistent behaviours to stress, nervousness, and stress. Meditation relies on an appreciation for the interconnectedness of all facets of the being, also attempts to unite and incorporate the vast array of factors that influence our wellbeing. In its core, the practice is a thorough method for self-development and conversion.

Yoga Supplies an Assortment of methods for recovery, Such as:

Postures: Yoga poses Help extend and strengthen your entire body and therefore are grounded in working principles which instruct proper posture and healthful body mechanisms. Becoming powerful, supple, and also nicely aligned improves your body's capability to satisfy the challenges of everyday life with ease in addition to its capacity to release stress, improve circulation, and improve energy circulation.

Breathing Practices: At a civilization where Folks tend to be shallow"chest Breathers," learning how to breathe deeply and completely offers excellent physiological and mental advantages. Bringing down air to the bottom part of their lungs, where oxygen flow is the most effective, causes a cascade of modifications heart rate slows, blood pressure decreases, muscles relax, nervousness eases, and the brain melts. By comparison, chest breathing may cause, or aggravate, neck pain as it uses accessory respiratory muscles around the neck, like the scalenes, to raise the torso, making compression to the thoracic spine (see chapter 2, figure 2.3, such as instance of the region).

Mindfulness: Meditation is a training Of consciousness that instructs us to be within every moment and to be within our own bodies. This may be a significant struggle in our contemporary world, where folks have a tendency to dwell in the mind when dismissing signals from the remaining portion of the human body to the degree that the human body has to yell in pain to find attention. Yoga counters this inclination to reside in the neck up by assisting us join our bodies and minds throughout the breath. The practice invites us to attract our focus , comprehend where we routinely hold stress and learn how to launch it.

Meditation: a Lot of Us often possess chattering thoughts continuously rattling about in our minds: What is next In my to-do listing? Can I turn off the cooker? I wonder what is on TV tonight? That is a state of chronic mental busyness that lots of meditation instructors call"monkey mind" Meditation is a powerful tool for calming the cluttered brain, enabling us to discharge distracting (and frequently stress-provoking) ideas and also to bring our awareness and attention to the current moment.

These diverse tools Operate in a synergistic manner. In his novel, Yoga as Medicine, Dr Timothy McCall (2007, 4) writes,"You stretch and strengthen your muscles, which impacts blood circulation, digestion, along with breathing. You relax and fortify the nervous system; also, it impacts the mind. You cultivate reassurance, and it affects the nervous system, the immune system, and the circulatory system. Yoga claims that in case you look obviously, you are going to understand that everything about you're linked to everything else."

Therefore it should come as no real surprise to find out that yoga tutors do not simply tell their customers,"Require this particular pose and call me in the daytime " Assessing bodily postures can be immensely beneficial in relieving and preventing neck pain as well as other disorders, buttrue recovery entails both everything you are doing to the mat and the way you live your own life. In case the moment you depart from your yoga mat, then you start to slump and tense your shoulders, then you are going to earn less progress in relieving your neck pain compared to if you attract the teachings of yoga into your daily pursuits. By way of instance, focusing on standing and sitting with good posture during your day; with a headset rather than holding the telephone between your ear and shoulder and getting slow, deep breaths when you are feeling stressed are fundamental methods to incorporate yoga exercise in your daily life.

Yoga Also teaches that it is not merely exactly what you can do, however just how you get it done that is crucial. Contrary to the Western practice mindset that states that the harder you work, the more

Better the outcome, in yoga we frequently go Quicker, maybe not by working tougher however by"playing milder," a curious way to the practice which reinforces the capacity to unwind, discharge, and go ahead. Yoga encourages one to equilibrium effort and concede, guts and care --to battle yourself however never pressure. In yoga training, learning the way to"reverse" is as significant (and for many people longer significant) as learning how to"do." (See chapter 5,"The way to Exercise.") Instead of muscle your way to a yoga posture, you learn how to relax to itusing the resources of patience, gravity, along with the breath--to permit the pose to weaken and unfold.

Over the years, with Normal practice, the lessons learned about the yoga mat start to affect how you reside on the planet. When your boss comes booting into your workplace with an urgent mission, rather than engaging on your habitual response of jelqing your spine and gritting your teeth, then you might end up reacting by pausing to have a deep, slow breath and consciously relaxing your shoulders. When turbulence starts to rebound the aeroplane you are flying , you might shut your mind, turn your focus to a breath, and start extending your exhalations to calm your body and head. Yoga teaches you how you can relax and breathe because you put yourself into hard positions around the mat so when you end up in tough positions in everyday life, you may draw on those skills to help keep yourself balanced and wholesome.

Assessing the Proof

Western Practical research to yoga's therapeutic advantages is comparatively fresh, but it is flourishing --with over a million studies requiring yoga recorded from the National Library of Medicine's analysis , PubMed (www.ncbi.nlm.nih.gov/pubmed). Posted in the USA, over sixty-five federally and privately supported practical trials are underway analyzing yoga's benefits for an assortment of ailments, including sleeplessness, cardiovascular failure, gastrointestinal headaches, epilepsyand diabetes, obesity, and hot flashes, arthritis, and post-traumatic stress disease, along with cigarette dependence (PracticealTrials.gov, www.practicealtrials.gov, s.v.,"Yoga"). Along with also an emerging body of literature indicates that yoga may alleviate a vast variety of ailments, such as chronic low- back pain, hypertension, irritable bowel syndrome, menopausal and perimenopausal symptoms, depression, stress, fibromyalgia, carpal tunnel syndrome, and also obsessive-compulsive disorder. Yoga's impact on neck pain has not yet been the subject of printed scientific research, but powerful evidence for yoga's efficacy in alleviating back pain provides confidence that research may finally Encourage yoga as successful self-care for neck pain Too (Sherman et al.. 2005).

One clear advantage of Yoga that many experts agree is the way it can ease stress, which is very important because 60 to 90 percent of all physician's office visits from the USA are stressassociated (Benson 1996). Stress has been demonstrated to possess wide-ranging consequences on mood, emotions, and behaviour. In her book, Self-Nurture (2000, 28), pioneering mind-body medication specialist Alice D. Domar notes that"chronicstress can activate continually substantial levels of stress hormones (as an instance, cortisol and adrenaline) that create elevated blood pressure or heartbeat, increased oxygen intake, diminished immune systems, along with physiological ailments that eventually cause symptoms as well as full-blown ailments." Domar calls for yoga a"powerful strategy...for relaxation and reinvigoration of body and mind"), also writes that a lot of the patients"report which yoga is one of the best stress-relieving methods they have ever practised".

Therapeutic Yoga

Yoga Is used in modern practical settings as an adjunct treatment for a wide variety of health issues --from heart ailments into hot flashes. Some pioneering medical facilities (like Duke Integrative Medicine, at which I practice yoga treatment), practices, and personal studios offer you individualized yoga sessions called yoga treatment . In such one time sessions, then a yoga therapist adjusts the practice to fit your particular requirements, developing an individualized yoga course made for practice in the home. Normally, this entails yoga poses, breathing exercises, and relaxation methods. Yoga therapy may be especially valuable for men and women that are not able to take part in a standard group course or who have particular issues, like fibromyalgia, hypertension, or asthma. The objective of the sessions is to enable you to advance toward better health and well- being.

Additionally, a growing number of hospital-based health centres Provide yoga Courses for overall well-being, in addition to yoga classes made for certain classes, for example, breast cancer survivors; individuals with MS, cardiovascular disease, and chronic pain; and teens with eating disorders. Therapeutically oriented yoga courses are often according to a gentle fashion of yoga.It's important to realize there are lots of unique schools and types of yoga--including a few that are rather challenging. By way of instance, Ashtanga yoga is quite athletic, whilst Kripalu yoga will be milder.

It is nice to attend A yoga course to match your practice on this novel, as

Long since the course is proper for You and can be educated by an experienced and seasoned yoga teacher. Regrettably, yoga's flourishing popularity has led in Some classes which are known as yoga but are now"yoga-flavoured" workout Classes taught by teachers whose training includes attendance in a Weekend yoga workshop. (See the tools section for assistance locating qualified Yoga education

) Should you attend a sizable group yoga class that is too rough for your Particular fitness centre or one that is taught by a badly trained or Experienced teacher, you May risk harm. Request Prospective teachers how long They have taught yoga, in which they analyzed, and also, equally important, how long They have practised yoga and if or Maybe not they have a personal yoga practice. Authentic yoga education is suspended in A teacher's own yoga training, and also the ideal yoga instructors reside their yoga on And away from the mat. A proficient yoga teacher may never be a drill sergeant but may act as a facilitator--pointing out you From the management of your "internal genius " (instructor) and assisting you to research what works better for you personally.

The heart of the practice

Though yoga practices have been made to boost well-being, yogic tradition does not see improved wellbeing as an end in itself , instead, as a standard required to correctly connect with the soul. The ancient yogis believed disorder to be a barrier to enlightenment. In the end, it is hard to sit in meditation and combine with the heavenly when you've got a headache or a stiff neck. Similarly, if disease or even sedentary habits have left you too feeble and rigid to sit down relaxationably, yoga poses and breathing practices will be able to allow you to become healthier and strong enough to sit quietly and meditate. Your system is thought to be a temple of the spirit, and yoga exercise helps preserve this valuable vessel.

The attention of yoga training is to calm your mind. The

Yoga Sutras of Patanjali, the text which puts on the instruction of yoga at 196 succinct aphorisms, says:"Meditation is the limitation of the changes of consciousness."

Considering that a calm, secure mind is vital to well-being, many resources of yoga are designed to help calm your brain and harness its power to get physical, emotional, emotional, and spiritual recovery.

After the body and mind are calm, it is significantly easier to hear that"still, small voice" of their centre. As it is Hard to view the bottom of a lake Once the atmosphere is annoyed by end --which makes the oceans choppy and preoccupied --it can be tough to connect with our soul Once We're emotionally and physically restless. But when everything becomes calm and calm, we could see clearly into the base of the lake and also into the innermost recesses of the heart.

From the yogic tradition, the soul is frequently called our"authentic self" or even"supreme character." These teachings maintain our souls are equally --and they're formless, immortal, and merry.

CHAPTER TWO

❧

BREATH

In the conventional terminology of yoga, one word implies both energy and breath: prana. This isn't a coincidence. Each breath, also by providing the Body using oxygen, also encourages all that you do and what that the body needs. However you're breathing, your own breath is currently linking you to lifetime. You're able to think about each inhalation and each exhalation for a healing action that requires very little hard work without a prescription.

Your Breath is also the part of a pain or stress reaction that's the simplest to consciously alter. There is no simple means to consciously obstruct the transmission of a pain signal from 1 brain cell to the next or request your adrenal glands to quit releasing hormones. It's possible, however, readily learn how to slow down or exaggerate your breath. It requires little over a little focus on the breath. Modest changes in your breathing may result in large changes in the way in which the body and mind feature, such as reducing stress hormones and lowering your sensitivity to pain.

The Type of breathing Changes that disrupt an stress or pain reaction do not need learning how to manage your breath or carry out some other acrobatics of their lymph system. These methods are easy and relaxational and can be carried out anywhere, anytime. Studies have shown that just focusing on the symptoms of breathing can reduce tension and make you feel better (Arch and Craske 2006). The availability of this breath causes it the ideal place to start altering the chronic pain cycle.

In this chapter, you may Find out More about why breathing Is this important instrument for relieving pain. You'll also find three distinct kinds of yogic breathing techniques: (1) breath consciousness, (2) preventing the breath through gentle stretching and movement, and (3) breathing methods for relieving tension and pain.

Breathing is really a two-way street between Body and Mind

What happens to a breath after you Are below a great deal of stress? Whenever you're in pain? If you have never seen, start to listen. You'll certainly realize that the breath is just one of the very first places pain and stress appear.

The yoga tradition includes Long realized your breathing reflects that the condition of your body and mind. After the human body and head are bothered by stress, anger, sadness, sickness, or melancholy, the breath gets upset. For many people, stress and pain result in keeping the breath, breathing shallowly, or difficulty with breathing. This really is a timeless withdrawal reaction, together with the entire body seeking to shield itself from that which is stressful or painful. For many others, stress and pain cause quick breathing and maybe even hyperventilating. This really is a timeless emergency response, together with the entire body grasping to get the energy that it believes it must fight or flee a hazard. You could realize your breath follows the two routines, based on the form of stress and pain.

These modifications Are a standard and instinctive portion of the means by which the body reacts to guard you from bodily or psychological stress. Normal, obviously, does not necessarily mean healthy. If you're chronically under pressure or in pain, then these breathing patterns may become the standard. That can be less than perfect, as the exact same breathing patterns which reflect strain and pain additionally fortify strain and pain. Additionally, they disconnect you from your organic flow of prana and may hinder your body's capability to supply you with the energy that you want.

It does not need to be. This manner. It's possible to learn how to consciously relax your breathing whenever you're in pain or under pressure. If your breathing is relaxed, then your nervous system gets the message that you're safe also. This message exerts a cascade of changes within your own body and brain that may block or disrupt a complete crisis pain-and-stress response. The outcome is that you feel better while still instructing the body and mind a much healthier approach to react to stress and pain.

Working with the breath to change your Frame of Mind and body

The two-way link between the way you Breathe and the way you believe was demonstrated in a study which observed the way the breath obviously affects during happiness, anger, despair, and stress (Philippot, Chapelle, along with Blairy 2002). The researchers triggered those four emotions in participants and quantified the changes in breathing speed, depth, motion, and stress, and other facets of the breath. They discovered that there have been feature changes for every emotion. Joy, by way of instance, was correlated with smooth, steady, slow, profound, and relaxed breathing. Sadness, by comparison, was linked to irregular, shallow, and also stressed breathing interrupted with sighs and tremors.

In Another study, the Investigators switched the observations for every emotion to breathing directions. They'd participants alter their breathing

According to these directions, with no sign, the breathing patterns have been linked to certain emotions. The analysis discovered that the breathing routines faithfully created the feeling that they had been correlated with, with no additional emotion trigger or cue.

These studies and many others like them, affirm. What you could find yourself As you attempt the breathing techniques within this chapter. The breath is a powerful instrument for breaking the cycle That strengthens chronic pain and stress. When you Learn How to breathe in a Manner That supports feelings of relaxation, security, and Joy, it's possible to actually opt for these Experiences over anguish.

PRACTISING BREATH

Hands-on Breath

Notice the motion of the breath and outside of this Body and the motion of the body as you breathe.

Exercise:

Anytime To concentrate on health, health, and also the delight of being alive.

During stress or pain, episodes to change attention and also to find a Feeling of Security, management, and increased relaxation.

For as Little as 1 minute, so long as wanted.

You understand that you're breathing. But do you believe your own breath? Can you believe that the breath Since it enters and leaves your body through your mouth, nose, and stomach? Would you believe the motion of your stomach as you inhale and exhale? Breath awareness isn't anything more than that: the practice of discovering how it feels to breathe.

While it sounds easy And maybe not too intriguing, the longer you focus on the breath, the more you'll discover. By emphasizing the sensations of the breath, then You're learning how to select which senses to cover

Focus on in your system. This ability can be valuable once you're in pain. Even though the brain is automatically attracted to pain senses, it may be hard-pressed to pay additional attention to other senses. This creates breath sense exceptionally soothing to the body and mind.

Getting started

Breath awareness can be practised in almost any respect, but you could see that a relaxational seated posture is the most useful for keeping you focused. It's possible to sit upright in a seat or cross-legged around the ground, utilizing a pillow beneath the hips for assistance.

Breathe naturally With no attempt to restrain the breath, then breathe deeplybreathe"better" in any manner. You are not hoping to achieve anything except comprehension, and there's not anyone right approach to breathe. When you become aware of the breath, then you can discover that the level of your breath varies. It may slow down or overheat. It may just sense much easier to breathe. Permit any of them to take place naturally, with no strain or attempt to make it occur. In the event you encounter the reverse and discover paying attention to this breath is more stressful, you can quit at any moment.

The directions below Will encourage you to detect certain senses of breathing. The very first time you read the following directions, try out each proposal as you proceed. Research exactly what you believe, allow your attention rest on such feeling for several breaths and continue on to some other feeling when you prefer. You are getting to understand your breath and also everything it feels like to breathe. This very first time is similar to perusing a menu and having to taste just a sample of what before you purchase.

Following This first Read-through, but the very best method to practice breath consciousness is merely to shut your eyes and notice what you find. You'll have a sense of all the sorts of things it's possible to listen to, and also you do not have to run some checklist down. Simply direct your focus on the way it feels to breathe. Let's feel that the organic flow of energy linking you into life.

With Normal practice, you'll realize that particular sensations (such as your stomach enlarging or the sensation of the breath entering and leaving the nose) function best to calm mind and give you back home for your physique. After that, you can opt to concentrate only on these senses when you exercise breath consciousness.

Notice how the breath moves in and out of the body

Start by discovering each Breath as it occurs. As you inhale, then detect that you're inhaling. When you exhale, see that you're exhaling. You may say on your mind"inhale, then exhale" to remain concentrated. Continue this till your focus settles smoothly and gently about the breath.

Now notice If you're breathing through your nose or your mouth. See the breath entering and leaving your system and feel the feeling of the breath going through your mouth, nose, and neck. Notice if you are feeling any strain in the neck, neck, mouth, or facearea. If you do, encourage them to unwind. Can there be some noise into your breath? If that's the case, can it be an outside noise (one which others could listen) or an inner audio (one which only you may listen)? When there's a noise, listen for it for a couple breaths.

Notice how the body moves with the breath

Now put your hands on your stomach. Notice what's occurring as you breathe. Would you believe that the stomach expand as you inhale and contract as you exhale? Would you believe the motion of the stomach through your palms? Would you believe it from the stomach , as the stomach skin and muscles elongate about the inhalation and sequence about the exhalation?

Next, put your palms In your rib cage and also detect the method by which the rib cage goes together with all the breath. Would you believe the ribs contract and expand? Be patient. Take the concept which you're able to breathe where you put your palms. Let your hands listen to any feeling of motion. Then change your consciousness into the senses at the rib cage . Feel that the ribs expand along with the skin and muscles elongate because you inhale. Feel them contract and then draw as you exhale.

Now put a hand in your own Torso and notice the way the chest goes together with all the breath. Would you believe the tender growth of your chest as you inhale the autumn of The torso as you exhale? Do you sense it equally at front of your hands and at the chest itself? See the feeling of the top ribs extending along with the lungs Growing interior them.

Ultimately, rest your palms everywhere that's relaxational. Notice that the complete motion of the breath and outside of the human body along with the entire motion of the human body as you breathe. Notice the senses of every breath in and out each breath. This is the link to energy that is overburdened. All you have to do is welcome this. By devoting your focus on your breath, you also provide your body consent to breathe in a manner that encourages relaxation and healing

Freeing the Breath

Moderate stretches and moves to discharge Tension from the breath.

Exercise:

Anytime To encourage wholesome breathing habits.

As a Standalone yoga session or in the start of a lengthier session.

A complete practice will require five to Ten moments; individual stretches could be carried out individually for a shorter practice.

Among the best things, You can do to help your regular well-being will be know to breathe with less strain and effort. Tension at the breath may fortify stress and pain, but a relaxed breath sends a constant message into your body and mind that you're safe also. Releasing tension from the breath will allow you to breathe deeply and easily with no excess work.

Where does stress in The breath come out of? The majority of the time, it comes out of chronic tension within the human entire body. If you hold tension from the stomach, chest, back, shoulders and neck, the pure activity of your breathing lungs and muscles is limited. After the stomach, chest, back, shoulders, and neck are free of unnecessary strain, the organic breath is discharged.

Gentle stretching is The perfect approach to publish the breath. To achieve this, think of what it takes to blow a balloon up. When you choose a brand new balloon from a bag, it has not been stretched. If you attempt to split it, then you will fight -- there is too much immunity. Though you're working hard, the balloon doesn't fully match. But if you just take a few minutes to stretch out the balloon and try to inflate it, then you'll find it a lot easier to expand. Your human body and breath are the exact same manner: when you release the outer immunity (muscle strain), the breath may"inflate" you far less effort. Your expertise will be of a deeper breath with increased simplicity.

Freeing the breath Requires just a couple of minutes, but it's a strong effect on both body and mind. This makes freeing The breath that a ideal standalone practice to begin every morning or as a break in the office to give up the stress that builds up on Daily. It's also a Superb way to Start a longer Yoga training.

GETTING STARTED

The next set of easy Moves and moves can allow you to give up tension that limits the breath. The very first time you attempt those moves, you may use these to detect where you routinely hold tension on your breath. Before and after every stretch, put your palms in the human body where the stretch is designed to publish the breath (as revealed in the pictures). Inhale and exhale at an organic but individual manner. Do not attempt to induce a deep breath. Notice if this region expands and contracts as you inhale. Does this feel fluid together with the breath or suspended?

If following a few breaths, You really do not feel any motion in any way; it's a fantastic indication that you're holding tension within this field. Stretching and lightly moving this region can help to release the pressure, allowing the region to expand when you inhale. After extending this region, wait to see whether there's more movement within this area if you breathe. If this is so, this is a fantastic practice for you to exercise frequently.

In case you do not detectany change, and there's still no movement with the breath, so try imagining this part of the human body is calming and enlarging because you Inhale and discharging as you can exhale. Imagination is a powerful tool if attempting To alter the customs Of your entire body or mind; also, it needs no force or fight.

OPENING THE BELLY AND LOWER BACK

Spine wave

Releases: Tension from the stomach and rear.

Inhale: Proceed right into a front-body stretch By

drawing back your shoulders to lift your torso and yanking your back to your system to marginally arch the spine. The action of inhaling should make the move easier and deepen the stretch that you are feeling from the chest and stomach.

Exhale: Proceed right into a back-body stretch By drawing on the torso and belly into round the back and extend the spine. The action of exhaling should make the move easier and deepen the stretch you're feeling on your spine.

Why is this a Breath-freeing exercise isn't simply the 2 stretches but the way you go between them with all the breath. Permit every inhalation or exhalation start the motion and draw you to the stretch, and also feel that the conclusion of the breath finish the motion and then weaken the stretch. Locate a organic rhythm of shifting between both stretches along with your own breath.

Replicate for five to ten breath intervals.

Seated forward fold

Releases: Tension at the trunk.

Lean forwards at a seated posture --just As much as is more relaxational --and remainder on your own arms, a cushion, or anything service is offered to cut. Breathe easily and break. Feel the motion of breath on your stomach and backagain.

Stay for five to ten breaths.

Following the back wave and forwards fold, then return to sitting. Bring your hands on your stomach and feel that it grow as you inhale and contract as you exhale. Take Pleasure in the motion of this Breath from the stomach and rear.

OPENING THE UPPER BODY

Chest expander

Releases: Tension from the Torso and shoulders.

Clasp your hands Supporting your back or hit behind you to continue to the back of a seat. Draw your shoulder blades together to start the chest. Locate the stretch directly where your upper arms match the torso. Feel the breath on your torso, and allow the breath extend you out of the interior. Envision the lungs and soul enlarging because you inhale.

Stay for five to ten breaths.

Neck stretch

Releases: Tension at the Shoulders and Neck.

Dip 1 ear towards The shoulder on that side by side Bring your hands to rest in your torso, right under the collarbone. Feel the subtle motion of the breath below your hand.

Stay for five to ten breaths.

Following the torso and Neck stretches, bring hands to break in your chest. Envision directing the motion of the breath To your palms. When you inhale, feel that the chest grow. As you exhale, Feel it fall. Then bring 1 hand into your stomach And texture both the torso and stomach expand as you inhale and inhale because you exhale. Take Pleasure in the motion of the breath In body.

Upper back stretch

Releases: Tension at the upper shoulders and back.

Clasp your hands in front of you. Straighten your arms and

then press on the palms away from one to disperse the shoulder blades. Reduce your chin on your chest. Feel the motion of the breath from the upper back. Allow the breath extend you from the interior. Envision the lungs extending straight underneath the top rear ribs.

Stay for five to ten breaths.

After extending the top back, Give a kiss, crossing Your arms on your chest. Bring your consciousness to Your spine, and picture directing the motion of the breath into your spine. Feel The torso extend beneath your arms. Take Pleasure in the motion of the breath In the torso and body, believing both grow as you inhale and contract because you exhale.

OPENING THE SIDE BODY

Side stretch

Releases: Tension in the muscles of the rib cage And unwanted body.

Lean-to one side, Allowing the backbone and rib cage bend till you feel a stretch at your unwanted body. Support yourself in your own hands or elbow. Feel the motion of the breath from your side and allow the breath elongate you out of the inside out.

Stay for five to ten breaths.

After extending the side body, then bring 1 hands to sleep on the side knee or ribs

That you stretched. Imagine Directing the motion of the breath on a hand. When you inhale, feel that the side Body extend. When you exhale, feel that it deal. Take Pleasure in the motion of the breath From the opposite body. Repeat for the next side.

End in any relaxational place. Shut your eyes and revel in the feeling of your body going as you breathe. Notice the way your body feels with spent this time breathing and stretching. Did anything regarding your breathing switch from earlier this practice?

BREATHING FOR PAIN AND STRESS RELIEF

Breathe in the stomach, rib cage, And torso with a gentle grin on your face along with the picture of your soul enlarging.

Exercise:

Anytime to reconnect into the internal joy that is the true character. For ten breaths or provided that is required and useful.

The breath of pleasure is a Easy practice that could change your frame of mind by simply altering the standard of your breath.

Come to some Relaxationable vertical position, standing or seated. Put your hands over the heart, and then detect the organic motion of breath below your hands. Relax your head, neck, and shoulders.

As you inhale, feel The breath extend the lower stomach, upper abdomen, rib cage, and torso. Feel each region enlarge softly, like a tide which begins from the lower stomach and crests in your own heart. Be patient with every inhalation and maintain inviting the breath (without stress) till you feel full and glowing using breath. When you exhale, allow the breath move with no effort. You will possibly start your mouth and allow the exhalation be an simple, gentle sigh. Both inhalation and exhalation ought to be free of stress. Have the impression that you're getting each breath and warm it with a open centre. Maintain a gentle grin in your face.

Expanding and contracting, and into the Feeling of it contracting and expanding.

As Soon as You connect to the sensation of the breath, shut your eyes. Feel your heart centre, right under your palms. Picture one of these on your Heart centre: your heart, resting between your lungs; even a sunlight, glowing Brightly; or even a world of light on your favouritecolour. Envision it enlarging because you inhale and contracting as you go. Connect into the visual picture of it

The Relief Breath

Gradually extend the length of your Own Breath into Your Own four-count inhalation and eight- count exhalation.

Exercise:

Throughout pain or stress, episodes to Discover a sense of security, management, and Larger relaxation.

Provided that is required and useful, making certain there's not any strain or fight. Return to relaxed, Natural breathing when any distress or stress happens.

The aid breath may Help you get through pain episodes and psychological overload. This breathing system helps people find a feeling of security and control over not only chronic pain episodes but also fear attacks, medical processes, tumultuous flights, along with almost any sort of stress you are able to picture.

The aid breath reduces pain, distress, and stressIn two major ways:

1. By slowing down your breath Extending your exhalation, it activates the relaxation reaction and shuts down The emergency pressure reaction.
2. It focuses your mind on a thing easy to control. This creates a feeling of security that may make the brain and body sensitive To pain and threat.

Count the breath

The Second step of the relief breath is to earn the exhalation longer than the inhalation. Start to count the distance of each inhalation and exhalation. The exhalation might already be slower compared to the inhalation--for instance, you might depend on three as you inhale but find you can count to five as you can exhale.

Over many rounds of Inhaling and exhaling, proceed toward slowing down the exhalation down to two as long as the inhalation (for instance, inhale for four counts, then exhale for eight points). The key to this technique isn't straining and struggling on the exhalation and not gasping for a last breath on the inhalation. Be patient, and also just have the aim to exhale completely. If you breed to lengthen your exhalation, you will make more stress on your machine -- exactly the opposite of what the relief breath is meant to do. Don't force a 1:2 ratio if it doesn't feel comfy. If you can easily extend the exhalation simply by one count compared to the inhalation, or perhaps merely to equal spans of inhalation and exhalation, that's fine.

After You Discover a Steady rhythm, try inhaling and

exhaling through the nose only. If you can keep a gradual steady exhale and simple relaxed inhale with the mouth shut, continue. Otherwise, return to pursed-lip exhalations. Throughout the extended exhalations, imagine letting go of pain, stress, and anything else you do not need.

You Can continue the aid breath for as long as you'd like, but frequently the benefits come in the very first few moments of lengthened exhalations. If you end up holding your breath or forcing the breath, go back to relaxed breathing.

For a variant of the Relief breath that provides a healing meditation, you can use a yoga mantra (a recovery phrase) into"count" the inhalation and exhalation. Rather than counting To eight and four, you can use a more four-syllable mantra to the inhalation (for example, sa-ta-na-ma or omShanti om), and replicate it twice as your own exhale.

The Balancing Breath

Part 1 (Alternate Nostril Breathing): Move through right nostril, exhale through left nostril. Then inhale , go right. Continue alternating for ten rounds (twenty-five breaths). Return to relaxed, organic breathing when any distress or stress happens.

Part 2 (Visualization): Picture alternative nostril breathing for ten breaths. Visualize inhaling and exhaling through the ideal nostril and entire side of their human body for ten breaths. Switch to imagining inhaling and exhaling through the left nostril and entire left side of their human body for ten breaths. Switchback and on

Between left and right sides for Ten breaths. Breathe through the nostrils, imagining the breath going through the

---

entire body, including ten breaths.

Exercise:

Throughout pain or stress, episodes to Discover a sense of security, management, and Larger relaxation.

In mattress (part 2 only) to conquer stress or pain-related sleeplessness.

The balancing breath Is especially valuable for reducing stress. Its Sanskrit title, Nadishodana, literally means"cleansing" This isn't only yogic legend--study has proven that this breathing technique may wash off the consequences of pressure, reducing blood pressure and heart rate (UpadhyayDhungel et al.. 2008; Srivastava, Jain, also Singhal 2005). As you exercise the balancing breath, then you'll discover that it instils reassurance and a feeling of ease within the human body.

Getting Started

To Start, draw your hands into place as shown: stretch all five hands, then fold your hands and middle fingers in toward your hands. That leaves your thumbring, and pinky fingers extended. You may use the rule to close your right nostril and your ring and pinky fingers to close your left nostril.

Attempt This today --bring your hands into your nose, and then exercise closing the ideal nostril with your palms. Notice the way you can still breathe during your abandoned nostril. Then discharge, and exercise Shutting your left nostril with your ring and pinky fingers. Notice how you can still breathe through your right nostril. Keep your mouth shut, and breathe Only through the uterus for the remainder of this practice. If this is tough Because of congestion, forget the very first portion of the practice and exercise just Part 2, that the visualization.

part 1: alternate nostril breathing

Inhale through both nostrils, then close the left nostril and exhale through the ideal nostril. Inhale through the ideal nostril, then close the ideal nostril and exhale through the left nostril. Inhale through the left nostril, close to the left nostril, and exhale through the rightside. Continue alternating in this manner for fourteen days (twenty-five breaths).

As you exercise, try to create every inhalation and exhalation about in span without pushing or straining. Have an awareness of patience with all the breath. Permit each inhalation and exhalation to become slow, stable, and eloquent as is comfy.

Following your closing Exhalation, relax your hands in your lap. Inhale and exhale through the nostrils for many breaths

part 2: alternate nostril breathing visualization

For ten breaths, shut your eyes and envision alternative nostril breathing. Keep your hands relaxed on your lap. Imagine inhaling through the ideal nostril and exhaling left. Imagine inhaling through the left nostril and exhaling right. Continue this manner. Do not fret about if you're really breathing in and outside only 1 nostril. Simply connect to this thought and feeling of the stream of breath.

Subsequently, for ten breaths, then Remain with the ideal side of their human body. Imagine inhaling and exhaling through the ideal nostril only. As you do that, imagine the breath flowing into and from the entire right side of their human body. When you inhale, imagine the breath flowing to the ideal side of the heart, your shoulder, arm, and hands; your best hip, leg, and foot. Envision the breath flowing back from the entire side of their human body. Connect to this feeling of the entire side of the human body .

Now change to the left side. For the following ten breaths, then imagine inhaling and exhaling through the left nostril only. Envision that the breath flowing into and from the entire left side of their human body. Connect into the feeling of the entire left side of their human body .

Finally, For ten breaths, change back and forth between left and right sides with every breath. For a single breath, then imagine breathing and from this entire right side of their human body. For another breath, picture breathing and from the entire left side of their human body. Repeat a few more rounds (around ten breaths), alternating left and right sides.

End by inhaling and exhaling through the nostrils and in the entire body. Feel the entire body . Feel the entire body inhale. Feel the entire body .

Breathing the Body

Imagine You Could inhale And exhale through various pieces of your body. Proceed through the full-body, such as any locations which are stressed or in circumstance.

Exercise:

Anytime To unwind or irritate the entire body.

Throughout pain or stress, episodes to Discover a sense of security, management, and Larger relaxation.

A full-body practice will require at least five to ten minutes.

Breathing your system is A visualization practice accommodated by the conventional custom of yoga Nidra (yoga) along with the entire body scanning practice instructed in Jon Kabat-Zinn's mindfulness-based stress reduction plan for those who have chronic pain (Kabat-Zinn 1990).

Start in any Relaxationablerelaxation pose, as revealed. Watch chapter 6 for other relaxation poses.

Put your palms on Your stomach and feel the motion of the breath. See the stomach rising and falling, and see the breath going in and outside of the human physique.

In this practice, you Will imagine you could inhale and then exhale through various pieces of your body--like your nostrils have been transferred into that portion of the human body.

Begin with your toes. Imagine You Could inhale and exhale through the bottoms of your feet. Envision the breath entering your body through the bottoms of your feet, and also leaving your own body through the bottoms of your feet. Notice any flaws in your toes. Imagine the feeling of breathing throughout your toes. Feel, or envision, that stream of energy at the toes as you breathe.

Now repeat this Visualization for some other pieces of the body: Your lower thighs, legs, and upper thighs. Your buttocks, lower back, mid-back, and back. Your stomach and chest. Your shoulders, upper arms, elbows and lower arms, palms. Your own neck. Your brow and the crown of the head.

After you get into an Place that feels stressed, unrelaxationable, or painful, do not bypass it. There are numerous things you can attempt this will make you feel relaxational.

First, remain together with the visualization, also guide the breath directly In the sensations of pain or distress. Imagine the breath is massaging or dissolving the pain and strain. Envision the solidity of this strain or pain relievers. Locate the distance Within the pain.

Secondly, try shifting your focus back and forth Involving the awkward area and also a more relaxational location. For a couple breaths, then breathe to the painful region; to the upcoming few breaths, then breathe into a different place. Shifting back and forth like that may teach the brain how to provide the unrelaxationable senses less priority. You're practising a wholesome type of diversion: deliberate altering of your attention whilst being pose within your own body.

When You've worked Your way during the full-body, let's feel that the breath enter your system through your mouth, nose, and neck. Picture the

Entire body getting the breath. Feel the entire body . Imagine the feeling of breathing through your entire body, as if the entire body were Softly enlarging since you inhale and contracting as you exhale. Feel, or envision, the flow of energy throughout your body.

CHAPTER THREE

❦

MAKING FRIEND WITH THE BODY

A Lot of People with Chronic pain begin to observe the entire body as a prison and also worry about doing it. It's at times such as this you may, such as Kate, wind up wishing you did not have a body in any way. Some individuals with chronic pain wind up in this type of struggle by using their body they even consider ending their own life. They simply can't bear to be inside this body in this minute and can't find any method to feel at home in their entire body.

Should you are feeling that this way, It's absolutely Vital That You take Measures to irritate your entire body, all. The meditations and hints within this chapter can help you do exactly that.

What type of connection do you have along with your entire body?

How can you explain a enemy? You may State being about him makes you uneasy. Whenever you're compelled to be together with him, you want you can get as far off as you can. You truly feel mad just thinking about him and everything he's done to youpersonally. You may be shocked and shocked at the way he's betrayed your confidence. You do not wish to bargain with him. You do not wish to listen . Should you listen to him, it's simply because you're on guard, attentive for any indication that he will hurt you. You translate what he does and says because more proof he cannot be trusted, and he will continue to harm you.

Does this clarify Your connection with your entire body? Even though it can be shocking to understand you have been enemies with your entire body, many individuals who have chronic pain do this way in their own body at least a few of the moment. If you do, then you're not alone.

What's the alternative? Consider how you'd explain an actual friend. For starters, you still are feeling relaxational . You're at home and free for yourself. Being puts you into a much better mood. When you have got a bad day or are too worried, you may feel a need to associate with her. You may depend on her to be there for you once you want her. In addition, you care for her well-being, and you are aware that you'd be there for her at a time of need. You like helping her. If she has a issue, you hear. You search to be able to make her happy. You promote her when she is down. You find the good within her, even if she can not. You're thankful for her and can not imagine life without her.

Does this seem like The way you are feeling about your own body? Or does it seem hopelessly different in the connection with your own body --so absurd that Youcan not imagine anyone believing like about his or her entire body?

It is not absurd, and it's possible. If You are reading this novel, there is at A portion of you who's looking after your own body with support and care. Have a moment to thank the a part of you and Let it read.

Why anger hurts

Anger, despair, disappointment, depression, and frustration are normal reactions to chronic pain,but normal

Does not necessarily mean helpful. Negative feelings --such as anger--have been hooked to the pain system also, for a lot of folks, will activate a pain incident or create pose pain worse. Fixing your body such as the enemy will deepen each pain-related samskara you've got: the stress, the stress, the necessity to be attentive to any indication of pain, as well as also the catastrophizing of each new pain incident. Anger gets in the way of the capacity to look after your entire body and immediately takes over your own capacity for pleasure.

Holding your own body just as It's will create every measure Toward recovery simpler. It is going to also go a very long way in creating the current instant, despite pain, even more comfy. The urge to be rid of pain and disrelaxation doesn't need rejecting your physique. You can't walk away from the relationship with your entire body, however much you really are feeling threatened by it or need to deny it. As complex as modern medicine isalso, it has not yet figured out the way to exchange within a body you do not need to get a brand new one.

There Is a Great opportunity. You will, sooner or later in the future, maintain less pain. But there isn't any alternative to the life within the human body at this time. If you would like to lower your disrelaxation, then you can't wait till your pain has been gone to irritate your own physique.

Friendliness for a basis for yoga training

Each the yoga practices within this bookAre supposed to assist you to find a way back to seeing your own body as a serene and secure place to become. Yoga, even when practised with a mindset of self-compassion, can help you regain a feeling of being at home in the own body, even if you're having pain.

I encourage One to decide on a base of friendliness before beginning the yoga movement practices in the chapters which follow. Especially once you've got a background of pain, then yoga calls for a friendly disposition toward your own body. In yoga, you may meet physical limits and experience powerful senses.

It requires empathy toward your own body to understand how to respond intelligently to those struggles. You Have to learn how to manoeuvre your body With both guts and self-care. You do not wish to prevent possibly healing movement since you're fearful of getting hurt, but you also don't wish to push disrelaxation since you're determined not to be held back through pain.

By Way of Example, you will need to work out the distinction between a feeling that indicates actual threat -- allowing you know you ought to come from a stretch along with a feeling that only lets you Understand that some sort of modification is occurring at a stretch. You won't be able to get this done should you strategy yoga feeling stressed or upset regarding the limits of the entire body. Without initially setting a base of friendliness on your own body, you can end up so frustrated with any constraints or distress that you simply give up and lose out on the healing potential of motion. If you're utilized to dismissing the senses of the body, you might end up decided to push any pain that you are feeling, which will only irritate your stresssamskara.

It Is Going to also be Very Hard for you to devote to some

yoga practice If You're in Warfare with your physique. Befriending your own body --and always coming back into an awareness of empathy, nurturing, support, and also gratitude to your own body --will motivate you to make time to the yoga practice. You'll also find it less difficult to find out which yoga practices would be helpful for you. This will direct you when you build a private yoga program that's most therapeutic for your body and mind.

Taking Measures to befriend Your Own Body

The practices which follow will guide you in empathy, gratitude, And approval of the entire body. They're also an invitation to detect the way you think about, discuss, listen to, and see to your entire body in daily life.

All these practices Request you to encourage emotions and ideas on your body; you might not Have needed for a certain time. You Don't Want to, nor if you attempt to, push other feelings About your own body which might be a lot more relaxational at the moment. Whilst you start those practices, provide yourself permission To feel fuller and despair, Empathy and frustration, anger and ignorance --at precisely the exact same time If needed! When negative thoughts and feelings come up, simply see them and keep to Actively invite in feelings and thoughts of compassion and gratitude. This is a fantastic approach to use, not only in meditation, but if you end up suffering from anger, frustration, or despair about your own body or your own pain. With time, You Will Discover the mindset of Friendliness more organic, and it'll become a part of your subconscious, instinctive manner of relating to your physique.

The Practices

Body Gratitude

Reflect on distinct pieces of your body together with appreciation and gratitude.

Exercise:

Anytime to fix your connection with your physique.

Whenever you're feeling frustrated by illness or pain, or critical in your entire body, to consciously select friendliness on your entire body.

Following a health appointment, to remind yourself that your system is over its own diagnoses and symptoms.

A complete practice takes five to eight minutes; however, you can exercise the gist of this manifestation anytime simply by depriving yourself of one motive you're thankful to your entire body.

So when was the last time you ever felt sympathy to your physique?

For most individuals who have chronic pain, the phrase"body reacting" can appear perplexing, and even foolish. Gratitude for that?

It is possible, to begin with the easy actuality that this figure is the companion with this life journey. It must be appreciated and recognized for the way that it's transported you to the moment and let you experience all leading up to the instant.

This gratitude practice is an chance to reflect on the way

the system has affirmed you. Your body isn't different from the own courage, your strength, or even your own trip through life. It's your company, your house, and the tool where your life has been expressed. Whatever experiences and strengths, you're thankful for you are able to use to treat your relationship with your physique.

To start this exercise, bring into some supported place, seated or lying downagain.

Have a minute to feel your entire body, such as any indications of pain or distress. You're able to take notice of those sensations without allowing them take over your entire attention. After that, see some part of the body which feels a feeling of ease or relaxation. It might become your stomach, your pinky finger, the bottoms of your feet, along with the stomach rising and falling as you breathe. It is irrelevant where that feeling of relaxation and simplicity is. As soon as you end up in touch with this feeling, remain with this for a couple minutes. Let your attention rest on the way that part of the human body feels.

Subsequently, one by one, then reflect on distinct pieces of your body together with appreciation and gratitude. Ask yourself,"How's this part of my body encouraged me ? How has it enabled me to take part in life" Begin with a different area of the human body which feels comfy in this instant and finally work your way around your system to an area which generally encounters pain. Some areas to think about are (but Aren't Limited to):

Feet

Thighs

Hips

Belly

Back

Torso

Core

Shoulders

Arms

Palms

Neck

Face

The sense organs: mouth, nose, and eyes, eyes

Your answers might be abstract or literal. By way of instance, the heart actually fuels the whole body, moving oxygen to each cell within the human body. This manner, the centre supports each activity you've ever taken. You may thank your centre for providing you the chance to experience every moment of your lifetime. Metaphorically, the heart sings with joy, expands with love, and pounds with enthusiasm. You may feel reacting to the centre for letting you experience every one of those feelings. Literally, your legs and feet allow you to stand and continue through life. Thinking symbolically, you may reflect on the days you've stood up for what you've thought in or how far you've come in existence.

Trust anything comes up, even though it seems silly or sentimental. If nothing springs to mind instantly, consider focusing on now. What's this region of your body performed now? Can it allow you to enjoy a meal? Flip the pages of the book? Smile and kiss your puppy? Even if now has been so hard you've been struggling to do anything, and you're alive. Can you concentrate on gratitude on the lungs, your heart, and each system of the human body that's supporting you at this time? Would you really feel gratitude for just how hard the body is working to encourage you and provide you the chance to experience this second?

Occasionally this meditation contributes to despair Together with gratitude, particularly

In the event, you end up thinking about things your body no longer could perform effortlessly. You could also end up feeling critical of a part of the physique. Let these feelings and ideas come and go without slamming them or rejecting them. Notice them, since they might be small flashes of this samskaras that contour your daily experience of the physique. Even because they appear from dependency, you may select to come back to the gratitude manifestation.

End this practise by bringing your consciousness back to your breath. Put your palms somewhere on your system at which you are able to truly feel the motion of the breath. Repeat to yourself,"Thanks for this particular breath. Thanks for this moment."

Compassion Meditation for the Body, Mind, and Spirit

Wishon your wellbeing, joy, peace, and liberty From anguish. Exercise:

Anytime To fix your connection with your physique.

When You're feeling frustrated by illness or pain, or

critical concerning Your own entire body, to knowingly select friendliness on your entire body.

Following a medical consultation, to remind yourself that your system is much more Than its diagnoses and symptoms.

Before starting any Kind of treatment, exercise, movement, or therapy, To remind yourself of your goal to watch over your body as well as yourself.

A complete practice will require five to ten minutes; however, you can exercise the gist of this expression anytime simply by repeating the words of the meditation after.

In this meditation, You may replicate a set of brief phrases that provide yourselfand your body--empathy. It's possible to read out the statements aloud or replicate them quietly on your thoughts.

Initially, you may feel as if you're just repeating the phrases without even feeling any real friendliness toward your physique. You might even feel inner immunity as you repeat the phrases. Do not be worried about it. This meditation may be curative, even in the event that you end up experiencing opposite ideas and feelings simultaneously. You currently have the seeds of friendship inside you; copying the words is a means to cultivate these seeds. With the time, the heart and mind will adhere to the words, along with your real adventure of friendliness will soon blossom.

To Start, bring Into any supported place, seated or lying down, such as some of these restorative yoga poses.

To connect with your own body, put your palms somewhere on the body where you are able to truly feel the motion of your breath, including your stomach or torso. As a gesture of empathy, you can rather place your palms on part of your system, which typically encounters pain, even if that is comfy.

This meditation has three phases. To begin with, direct the next fantasies toward your own body as though it were a beloved friend, utilizing the term"you" You might choose to steer them toward a particular portion of the body which undergoes pain.

"May you be fit " "May you be pleased."

"May you be free of distress." "May you understand peace."

Repeat this original Point as many days as you'd like, discovering any ideas or feelings which come up. Afterwards, steer these Very Same fantasies toward your self --mind, body, and soul --with the term"I." Take special care to believe That You're

Including your own body on your awareness of self.

"May I'm fit "

"May I Be joyful."

"May I'm free of distress." "May I know peace."

If You Discover it Hard to connect with a real feeling of empathy, you may begin this practice by visiting mind a individual or creature for that which you really do feel an intuitive awareness of compassion and care. Direct the fantasies to them , then let the sensation of empathy take you to the custom of compassion on your own.

Ultimately, acknowledge that the liberty You need in this instant to select health, joy, and peace, by replicating these statements:

"In this instant, I'm already healthy and whole." "In this instant, I'd like to be joyful."

"In this instant, I decide to be free Of anguish."

"In this instant, I'm at peace with my own body, mind, and current experience."

All these statements are Not confident affirmations or wishful thinking. They're acts of empathy for your entire body, mind, and soul. Meditation is the practice of switching away from anguish and toward your inborn capacity for wellness, intellect, and pleasure. Whether you understand or believe those statements to be accurate, offering them is a reminder that you've chosen this route.

You might have discovered that some part of your brain would like to assert that you're not yet healthy and complete and you can't be happy and in peace so long as you've got pain. Simply observe these ideas and feelings and the way they make you really feel.

With practice, you'll discover it is Potential to genuinely rest on your very own sincere compassion and well-wishes to get Yourself, including the human entire body. When This comes to pass, enjoy the sensation. Allow it to be an imprint In your body and mind. You are able to take advantage of this meditation everywhere, anyplace, to reconnect with this sense.

Listening to Your Body

Exercise:

Anytime to start up to the advice of your internal wisdom and your body.

When You'reFeeling Overwhelmed or confused with pain, stress, or disease, to select 1 thing that you can consciously try to look after yourself.

Before starting any Kind of treatment, exercise, movement, or therapy, To remind yourself of your goal to watch over your body as well as yourself.

A complete practice takes five to eight minutes; however, you can exercise the gist of this manifestation anytime by simply just taking a few breaths to centre your brain and then requesting your entire body,"Exactly what do you really want?"

Stress is not the sole Important sign in the entire body, but it sure could be the loudest. Whenever you have chronic pain, listening to a body may look like the very last thing in the world that you would like to do on goal --particularly in the event that you translate"listening to a body" because"devote all of your energy and attention into your pain."

That is Not exactly what this practice requests you to perform. Waiting for your body is all about allowing all of the other messages out of your body talk for you--those frequently overshadowed by ignored or pain in your endeavour to dismiss your own pain. Waiting for your body is all about giving your internal wisdom a opportunity to provide you some advice about the best way best to look after yourself.

This manifestation will Help you get in contact with the portion of you who wishes to cultivate your own body. Additionally, it provides your body's brains an opportunity to surface on your open, open mind.

Begin this expression With a couple minutes of silent rest. If You're in pain, then rest might not necessarily Feel calm. That is alright. Just support Your own body as best possible And permit yourself to feel what's occurring at this time. When pain is pose, permit yourself to see it. If hunger Exists, let To detect it. If fatigue is current, permit yourself to see it. This will indicate a definite change from the mindset Of simply getting your own body throughout the struggles of this day, to your willingness to obey your physique

MOVING THE BODY

Among the initial things that pain will Is suspend the entire body. Muscles tightenjoints , and the idea of physical activity can get overwhelming. When pain is persistent, you may begin to feel locked into a body which has lost its capacity to move with strength and ease.

Freezing in reaction to pain is a standard Protective urge, and lots of individuals with chronic pain prevent movement as they're frightened of damaging themselves. However, in the long term, preventing movement generally causes pain worse. Moderate exercise is a much superior way for shielding yourself from additional pain or lack of work. Research proves that the physical activities of yoga can decrease pain, improve functioning, and lower the demand for pain medicine for types of pain which frequently cause people reluctant to work out, such as chronic low back pain.

Yoga's strategy to Motion is a particularly excellent form of exercise for most people in pain. You can go at your own rate, pick the moves that feel great to you, and also devote the time required to understand how to earn your body a relaxational position to be. You won't have to stress, drive, or even compete to obtain yoga's benefits. Yoga was made to release the power which flows through you and also to reestablish the awareness of being at home within your entire body.

To Tap to the human body's natural healing energy, the yoga tradition has generated two kinds of physical exercise:

(1) holding the entire body in different poses (known as asanas), and (2) fluidly moving in and out of poses, and coordinating the motion with the breath (known as vinyasa). This chapter will teach you , using poses and moves demonstrated to assist individuals with chronic pain.

The yoga exercises in this chapter Can assist you:

Conquer physical strain and stress.

Boost Your own mood.

Publish the nervous system natural Pain-suppressing substances.

Regain energy and strength for everyday tasks.

Learn The way to obey your body's signs and treat your self.

With regular exercise, The drills in this chapter may spare the body from the grasp of chronic pain and also remind one of the organic joy of motion.

YOGA'S APPROACH TO MOVING THE BODY

Vinyasa, or moving your system together with the Rush, is the basis of motion . A very simple instance of vinyasa is raising your arms overhead as you inhale and lowering them as you exhale. Why don't you put this book down and attempt this motion today? When you inhale, lift your arms. When you exhale, reduce them.

The Trick to locating The Yoga --that's the reunion of mind, body, and soul -- in something simple is to completely combine the motion along with the breath. You organize the time of this motion and breathing precisely. Provided that you're inhaling, you still ought to be raising your arms, rather than simply holding up them. And so long as you're still raising your arms overhead, then you still ought to be inhaling. There's not any use in time when you're moving your arms holding your breath, yet there's not any use in time when you're breathing but not going. To put it differently, there's not any separation between the motion of the body and also the motion of breath and outside of your physique.

With this in mind, Try out the arm-lifting movement . Spread the motion of your arms over the whole breath and the whole breath outside. You might have to slow down the breath along with the motion to bring them all together.

Did the motion sense different this time? Maybe more deliberate and more hierarchical? Are you conscious of your breath along with your own physique? As you understand how to completely synchronize breath and movement, even easy movements will get powerful recovery meditations.

Asana, or even holding Poses, is what the majority of men and women think about when they hear that the term"yoga": irregular contours of the human body which are stored for anywhere from several breaths to a lot of moments. It might appear strange this to spare the flow of energy inside your body; you'd remain still. On the other hand, the outward stillness of the body provides you a chance to discover the internal stream of energy pose within the human body. In yoga, you do not need to produce a great deal of energy by running about and getting your heart rate up. Yoga recognizes the stream of energy is inside of you, moving by you as breath and feeling. Being in the poses helps you sense it.

Each pose is also an exercise to your mind. Your Goal in every pose is to not

Go deeper at a stretch or maintain a pose Longer and more. Your intention is to have peace of mind in poses which produce powerful sensations of elongate or need attempt to maintain. As you learn how to get reassurance in every yoga pose, you're learning how to meet virtually any obstacle with patience, courage, and existence.

Among the best ways to earn a yoga pose--or even some other hard situation-- not as stressful would be to concentrate on The senses of breathing. Breath consciousness calms the brain and also makes it possible to remain in contact with the way the pose is affecting the body. Therefore for asana in Addition to vinyasa, breath Is again the crucial ingredient which produces a yoga exercise recovery. You will see this rule as you Understand yoga's relaxation and Meditation practices. As you know each new practice, Make Sure You notice what Role breathing plays inside. A constant focus on the breath will be sure that every practice is infused with healing prana.

IS YOGA SAFE FOR YOUR MEDICAL CONDITION?

Yoga has been demonstrated to be useful for a broad selection of health care ailments, such as cardiovascular problems, cancer, diabetes, obesity, and HIV. Yoga continues to be utilized to help rehabilitation from operations, such as hip replacementsand knee arthroscopy, and spinal operations.

But that doesn't mean that each and every yoga pose or motion is secure for each state. Important surgeries into a joint could permanently lower its assortment of movement, but these constraints vary widely by operation and patient. Consult your physician or physical therapist what moves (if any) are contraindicated to your affliction. In case you've got uncontrolled hypertension or pressure-related eye ailments like glaucoma, inquire if motions that attract the mind under the centre (like in a position forwards fold) are secure for you. In case you have osteoporosis or spinal injuries, you ought to be particularly tender in poses which require significant backbone motion (like at an bend twist or hammering the backbone to extend the spine).

Regrettably, there Are no universally approved motion guidelines for particular ailments. But using a physician's advice and your willingness to obey your body's opinions, you may greatly lower your chance of harm from any sort of exercise.

Bear in Mind that motion Is only 1 part of a recovery yoga practice. Even if a few poses aren't Suitable to the system, you can still keep enrich and complete yoga exercise by such as breath, relaxation, and meditation.

GUIDELINES FOR MOVEMENT THAT HEALS, NOT HURTS

A Lot of People with chronic pain have damage Themselves in different kinds of exercise also are cautious of attempting something new, such as yoga. Yoga's misleading standing for needing a contortionist's flexibility does not help the issue. The reality is, any kind of exercise could be healing or harmful, based on the way you approach it. The yoga moves within this chapter are available to the majority of people. These guidelines can allow you to ensure your yoga practise alleviates rather than strengthens your pain. It's possible to apply these tips to some kind of exercise, to help you remain safe whilst remaining busy.

Balance Effort and Ease

You will have Approached different kinds of stretching or exercise with a mindset of 100% effort--move out, push yourself to your own limits. This strategy is more likely to trigger chronic pain compared to cure this, and in the slightest, it's a guaranteed one-way ticket to harm.

Rather than pushing to Your constraints, consider staying at a 50 to 60 percent attempt zone. You ought to have the ability to breathe easily, keep the integrity of your own form, and also place a grin on your face in almost any yoga motion or pose. Exert yourself only enough to satisfy the needs of a motion or pose, using the smallest amount of pressure within your entire body and head.

If You Discover yourself Maintaining your breath

straining to breathe, you're pushing harder than you want to. If it seems as if you're fighting with the pose instead of appreciating it, then take the attempt down a notch or break. Try it with more simplicity and less pressure.

Not only will doing Less create the motion easier to your entire body; however, you'll actually get. Remaining at 50 to 60 per cent attempt will provide you the power and relaxation to remain in a posture long enough to allow this to change the human body's customs and build power, balance, and endurance.

Pay Attention

Yoga Motion is healing since it reunites body and mind. Yoga isn't something that the body can perform while your brain is otherwise busy. Mindfulness-- paying attention to what you're doing as you can do it and how it seems to perform itunlocks the full advantages of a motion or pose. Mentally evaporating, in contrast, permits you to strengthen old customs, so strengthening stress and pain.

As you exercise a Pose or movement, actually pay attention to what it is you're doing and how it feels. Stay connected to a breath, ideas, sensations, and feelings. Let your entire body and mind encounter the motion and get its benefits.

This is particularly Significant if a pose generates powerful sensations within your system, such as the feeling of a profound stretch or the feeling of muscles functioning to encourage you. It's appealing to block those out sensations, particularly in the event that you've learned to do so with pain.

There's a subtle, changing boundary between the senses of positive change going on in the body in a yoga pose. If you're not actually paying attention to the way, the pose feels, secure and wholesome sensations could be misinterpreted from the brain as pain. This may trigger a stress reaction that raises pain and strain. On the flip side, if you dismiss senses that are accurate warning signals, you're in danger of injuring yourself. But should you keep interested in senses and ensure you are not pushing yourself, then you are able to find out to relax to powerful but secure sensations while protecting yourself against harm. In every pose, keep in mind a feeling of friendliness and caring on your entire body. When a pose is debilitating, come from the pose and break.

Practice the Law of Karma

In yoga Doctrine, karma only suggests that each action has consequences. This can be true for many yoga poses; however, the ramifications of a pose can fluctuate from person to person and from day-to-day. To continue to keep your yoga practice recovery rather than dangerous, you have to be a pupil of karma.

As you exercise, See the effect every motion or pose has in the human body. Would you really feel relaxational? Are you really trying to breathe or breathing readily? Are there some new sensations from your system --and in that case, are they really pleasant or painful? In the event you change anything about how you're performing the pose, how does this change the way the pose feels? Following the pose, can there be more nuisance or not? Were the pose release or increase tension within your system?

Being a pupil of karma also means paying attention to the

way you feel later in the day as well as the subsequent day. Are you currently in less or more pain? Can you feel less anxious? What's your energy? What's your mood? How can you sleep?

As you listen to the results of your practice, you are going to find out to make your healing practice and prevent poses or motions which are much less beneficial for you. This lesson can take over into other fields of life, assisting you to listen to your entire body and care for it with compassion and wisdom.

Use Your Imagination

One of yoga's most great insights to the body-mind Link is your power of creativity. Traditionally, the yogis thought that imagining a motion before really doing it ready the body and mind to the complete advantages of a pose day. It's possible to take advantage of this principle to earn any motion more hassle-free.

It may seem like wishful thinking, But there is nothing mysterious or absurd about it. Scientific research has confirmed that imagining that the motion disrupts the body to manoeuvre with greater ease, relaxation, and ability. When you envision a motion, you trigger the very same regions of the mind and pathways of the nervous apparatus required for this particular movement. Your muscles are prepared to relax or work as required. Imagining a motion during the time that you're relaxed will even prevent unnecessary strain, bodily strain, and disrelaxation during the actual motion. Imagining a normally debilitating motion as reflexology can also train the mind to encounter it less debilitating.

Before attempting A new motion, read the directions, examine the pictures, and picture it in actions. Then close Your eyes and envision how it will feel to perform the motion with elegance and simplicity. If You Discover any motion or pose uneasy, you can always close your eyes And envision practising it, pain-free and coordinated together with your breathing. Even In the event, you don't exercise the pose with the entire body; you'll be producing real recovery pathways From the body and mind. You can also use the yogic method of Imagination to some motion, from getting from bed to driving your bicycle, and also to some forthcoming situation which you're concerned about, by a medical Process to people speaking. Imagining the motion or scenario while Maintaining a relaxed breath and body may go a very long way in assisting You deal with the challenge if you confront it.

SENSATIONS TO WATCH

Safe yoga may create A wide selection of new and interesting senses: the gradually decreasing strain of a fantastic stretch; the stirring of muscles that you never knew you'd; the sensation of your breath hitting into areas you never knew that could breathe. Sensations enable you to learn in your own body, and seeing the sensations within your body is able to turn into a healing meditation at its very best.

You will find several Sensations, but that indicate it is time to run out of a pose and potentially prevent it in the long run. Come out of the pose and break if you are feeling some of the following senses:

Disrelaxation that Increases since you maintain a stretch. Stretches--in case you don't push inside them should get more, less, comfy as you maintain them.

Disrelaxation which increases from 1 yoga session to another --for example, a pose that felt nice yesterday feels uneasy now. This implies you might have overdone it, and your body needs a rest.

Any Sort of distress Or attempt, which makes it impossible to breathe easily and deeply. This implies that you are working too hard and also the own body is getting a stress reaction to the seriousness of the pose. The best approach here is don't to get more.

Any type of pain that's sharp or shooting. Any lack of feeling.

All these Senses are more consistent with harm compared to positive changes you need in the yoga practice. You could be pushing the pose or remaining too long at the pose, or that pose simply might not be curing for you at that stage in time.

Use your judgment along with Different senses, understanding that yoga is meant to feel great during the time you're doing this, not in any stage later on. If any yoga exercise allows you to feel worse, not better, then allow it to go and find a distinct practice which is suitable for you.

Be Consistent but Not Rigid

Do not make yoga Complicated or time-consuming you need to drive yourself to take action. Doing just a tiny bit of motion daily is far better than performing one hour once weekly. Carrying out a couple of minutes many times through the day is much better. Should you take the mindset that you Want to practice the Whole order Described within this chapter every time you Practice or invest a particular quantity of time in your own yoga each single day, you'll put up an unnecessary obstacle to performing yoga.

The main thing is to make yoga a regular part of the lifetime. You would like to produce a custom of being on your own body, and along with your entire body, at a healing manner. To assist this custom, take root, Start Looking for Five to eight minutes and there to manoeuvre your entire body, breathe, Stretch, and unwind. The sequence in this chapter Isn't a prescription that is fixed. It Doesn't Have to Be performed in the Purchase Introduced in its entirety, or even to get Any established time period. You can choose just a couple of moves or introduces And let them become a standalone practice. Any of these poses may be paired with a Favourite breathing, Meditation, or relaxation exercise to produce your very own mini-healing practice.

The sequence

The sequence that follows is quite a fundamental, well-rounded practice which includes poses and motions which were shown to assist individuals with chronic pain. The sequence is arranged to six pairs of energetic poses and one pair of three gentle poses to prepare one for relaxation. Every pair of busy poses signifies both the vinyasa(a constant stream between both poses) and introduces you may also practice individually.

A superb way to exercise the busy poses within this order would be to approach each set for a flow , moving between both poses with every breath. Subsequently, hold each pose for five to ten breaths before continuing on to another pair of poses. Consistently rest for a couple breaths between flows and poses. Utilize this opportunity to discover the impacts of the motion on your entire body, mind, and soul. This strategy maximizes the healing power of this sequence. The last three tender poses could be kept for five to ten breaths or more. Rush in those poses rather than attempting to work in them. Permit each pose to loosen some lingering strain within the human body and breath.

Each pose will consist of guidelines for actions --exactly what to do--and feeling, or exactly what to feel and notice. The actions guidelines help make sure the movement is secure. Follow the directions for every gift as you can. Then let your encounter from the pose --are you really comfy? In pain? Enjoying the pose?

--be the principal source of opinions about if you are performing the pose correctly. Sensation and breath will probably provide you the very best feedback about if a pose is secure and recovery for you.

Among the clearest indications that a pose isn't best for one (at least now) is if you encounter powerful unrelaxationable sensations which make it tough to focus on the breath and another senses recorded for every pose. While this occurs, attempt to alter the pose until it's relaxational enough, which it is possible to focus on the breath along with other recommended senses. If your expertise from the pose remains controlled by sensations of pain or stress, come from this pose, break, and try an alternate string.

It's possible to practice this order in the sequence. It's posed or construct a shorter practice based on what you require.

For every sequence, modified variants employing a seat for support will also be displayed. These seat versions give the very same advantages as the simple sequence but might be more pleasurable if you're interested in finding a practice that's gentle on the joints and offers additional support for balance and durability. You may also discover the chair variations for a Terrific Way to bring yoga to areas where it could be

Struggling to roll out a mat and then put around the ground. Straightforward seat yoga poses could be a terrific break in the workplace, in waiting rooms, and also in the airport. (Ignore any funny looks that you receive --the advantages via an impromptu yoga session really are really worth being a general function model for yoga!)

Everything You Require

A yoga mat (known as a"sticky mat" since it prevents slipping) is useful but not crucial. It's possible to practice on a different kind of workout mat, a tough floor, or even a rug, so long as you are feeling encouraged. A pad, towel, or blanket to your floor introduces will make you relaxational. You might want a sturdy seat near to try out a number of those seat variants. If you are interested in purchasing a yoga mat or cushions and blankets made particularly for yoga training, visit the tools section at the conclusion of the book.

Everything You Do Not Require

If at all possible, practice . Eliminate any watches, jewellery, or restrictive clothes that can interfere with your relaxation or breathing. In addition, I urge not practising facing a mirror on a standard basis. Even though it can be valuable to find some visual feedback when you're first learning poses, mirrors may take you directly from your own body's expertise and to self-criticism or diversion. Better to sense that the poses, from the interior, than invest your energy assessing everything you look like inside them.

WILL YOGA HELP EASE BACK PAIN

During time, there's been a great deal of debate with respect to what exactly would be the very best ways of alleviating back pain. It is a simple fact that there are varying degrees of pain at the trunk, and several back victims have a tendency to emphasise their spine, in addition to neglect to do things with the perfect body posture. A good deal of published medical journal studies; however, have agreed a very simple kind of yoga will do a whole lot to substantially alleviate the signs of pain.

The published studies have suggested that practising the easy kind of yoga will help to greatly alleviate back pain, in addition, to decrease the distress, stiffness and other relevant symptoms. It was mentioned that the people who attend yoga classes and perform so little as 75 minutes of exercise, also revealed significant progress in relieving the symptoms of back pain, even compared to individuals who did nothing in any way. The analysis also pointed out that even people who practised yoga in-home even revealed better outcomes, compared to individuals that attended formal yoga and workout courses.

The exercise courses were mostly designed by yoga instructors to specifically cover the issues of spine pain, and actions such as forwards stretches and assorted spins were undertaken by every student. Some exercise routines were also replicated, based upon each pupil's energy levels. All exercise participants nevertheless, manifested considerable advancement.

Yoga is proven to provide the body an assortment of advantages. It supplies suppleness and elasticity into a individual's body, in addition, to fortify the muscles and also re-balance your system. Because there are various kinds of yoga, pupils should be able to discover the perfect course and teachers to them. As soon as you start the yoga course, you should begin gradually, and also do things lightly, in addition, to maintain a open mind, and then follow along to the hilt exactly what your teachers say, after undertaking the exercises.

Yoga specialists worry the appropriate exercise regimen should begin with the ideal posture. The nasal tip is 1 exercise method that is frequently unnoticed facet but is frequently regarded as an essential cog in reducing back pain. Doing the pelvic tip will help considerably enhance and fortify the human body's core muscles, in addition, to further reduce strain on the trunk, and update the body total equilibrium.

A very simple core position is your Plank, either forearms on the ground or with arms directly. Keeping this position for 30 minutes or longer with just a tiny tailbone tilt provides strength to a heart and keep alignment.

It is often emphasized that yoga comes with an additional spiritual circumstance, and it's much more than only a mere exercise regime. Performing yoga exercises, including meditation and other relaxation techniques, can really greatly alleviate stress, in addition, to bring a calm and calming feeling to the individual. Most yoga urges agree that performing twenty-five minutes of meditation could be like sleeping for eight weeks.

People who suffer with back pain will be pleased to inform you that reliably practising the craft of yoga will do a fantastic deal in alleviating pain. Exercises like strengthening, toning and stretching contribute a whole lot towards drastically reducing pain. As individuals who suffer with this debilitating illness get to find out more about their own body, they will determine that stress plays a main role in ridding back pain. Faithfully following the tenets of yoga allows for a more holistic recovery procedure, which ought to do more than just eradicate a debilitating neck or back.

The philosophy behind yoga pressures you ought to proceed in a way that doesn't pressure or apply too much pressure on the body. Yoga ought to be a meditative kind of exercise and treatment, that ought to be practised in such a way that harmonizes all facets, such as brain, soul and body, and though it might appear hard to follow in the beginning, continuous practice ought to allow you to perfect your art.

As you keep learning more about the centuries-old method of yoga, then you are going to determine that the various postures and exercises can provide you greater insight in your own body's alignment. As we frequently spend the majority of our day sitting on a desk, working at a computer, and also invest just time working out, our joints and muscles weaken and do not properly work.

Normal yoga exercises helps refresh, realign and fortify our joints and muscles, improve our position, subtract our body equilibrium, and general relieve the pain caused back pain. With just a small effort, you're understand that doing a few moves, and frequently meditating, will perform a fantastic deal in twisting off the rigours of spine pain.

When we come in the centre in our practice, instead of in the self, the outcomes will probably be life improving. Our self encourages us, although initially to begin with that is OK, then our self pushes us farther. And when we don't control our self, we could wind up with more pain since we're working too hard! By maintaining inthe stream with the celestial', we shall reach more about a deeper degree.

For years, many medication and therapy modes are formulated to combat back pain, and many muscle relaxants and anti-inflammatory drugs are promoted as the significant cure for a debilitating back. A good deal of back pain victims also have been proven to only stay stuck, and suffer the pain caused by this disorder, possibly due to fear or ignorance.

The incessant distress caused by this illness can be really unkind to the individual, both emotionally and physically. Doing simple family or work-related activities may be a really hard one for pain at the back victims, and many patients are made to devote massive amounts of money for nonsurgical and sometimes addictive therapy types.

What is great about practising yoga is all that, there is considerable evidence to suggest that the meditation and exercise patterns of yoga help a great deal in reducing spine, shoulder and neck pain, too in rehabilitating and strengthening your body's joints and muscles.

There is a popular belief, which emphasizes that bed rest

is the ideal treatment for back pain. But, I must worry that maintaining the body going, in addition to maintaining the flow flowing by doing gentle exercises, so need to do more to alleviate back pain. Bear in mind which you will need to obey your entire body, in addition, to prevent exerting too much strain on it.

It is estimated that approximately 65 million people in America suffer with back pain, and should you chance to be among them; then you need to try getting yourself at a yoga course. Meditation is a meditative and relaxing type of exercise, which you will need to share in, irrespective of your age or ethnicity.

A good deal of research have revealed that yoga provides more advantages compared to other traditional forms of exercise daily. The relaxation exercises, meditation periods, breathing and stretching patterns of yoga are excellent at reducing strain on the trunk, shoulders and neck.

Undertaking a combination of yoga postures need to help align and strengthen the backbone, and so speed-up the human body's capacity to recuperate. If such exercises are done on a regular basis, you will make certain to relish long-term positive aspects, and shouldn't cover expensive and potentially addictive medical remedies.

Getting into a normal pattern of yoga practice is a fantastic habit to adopt. It's fantastic, to begin with, a brief period of exercise state, half an hour in the daytime and building up slowly to maybe one hour or even 1 and a half an hour. Most courses run for one and a half an hour. Try it and watch.

It's projected that approximately 80 million men and

women in the USA regularly look for treatment for shoulder, neck and back pain. At this speed, it'd be safe to state that just twenty per cent of Americans are now healthful and pain-free.

But, there's very good news for people who suffer with persistent back pain. Yoga that can be a revered thousand-year practice may be really helpful in treating back pain. Yoga is very good for physically emotionally and emotionally frees up you, and is good for relieving stress, and it has other associated impacts. When you have the ability to ascertain your programs, in addition, to take the time to exercise this revered kind of meditation and exercise, then locate a course that suits your schedule, and search for friends or friends who will join you into exercising.

Yoga is a really gentle and private way of attaining your own physical and psychological demands. When intentionally practising it, then it is going to help rejuvenate the senses, in addition, to cure any joint or muscular pains you might encounter. Based upon what you require, yoga can be practised in a fashion that fulfils your needs of your entire body and head, and you'll likely also get the job done too deep or as shallow as you see it all fit.

It is a simple fact that spending long hours seated in the desk or lifting heavy things the improper manner, may be detrimental to your spine, spine and neck. Whatever you are doing, keep your eye on your position. If you are sitting in your desk, then don't forget to keep your spine straight, rather than constantly being hunched or bending harshly. Spending a lot of time in your desk may lead to the shortening and depriving of your chest or back muscles, which may result in chronic back and shoulder pain.

To ease strain and stress, always execute yoga's stretching routines, exercise and meditation methods, so you'll have the ability to ease body pain. Daily exercise also helps in toning your aching and tired muscles, in addition to in massaging your joints. In case you've got a 9 to 5 desk job, consider quitting your desk for a couple of minutes, also spend some time doing short walking and stretching exercises, in addition, to devote substantial time throughout this nighttime, for practising the tenets of Pilates.

Maintaining the body cellular is essential and being conscious of your position; it does not require a lot to throw your body out of misery. Small and often through daily is a fantastic method to assist a wholesome body.

CHAPTER FOUR

☙

YOGA POSES FOR PAIN RELIEF

Sun Breath (Mountain Pose and Sun Pose)

Mountain pose

All these Poses connect one to the stream of energy and breath inside your system.

Start in: Mountain pose

Inhale: Sun pose

Exhale: Mountain pose

Mountain pose is a Chance to explore Pain-free posture and exude calm assurance.

Do: Stand straight with your feet hips-distance apart. Research how it seems to endure and locate your most relaxational posture. If you truly feel balanced and steady, bring your palms together in front of your torso. Close your lips or eyes in your palms.

Feel: The grounding of the feet, the Symmetry of the entire body, and also the motion of breath wherever your palms join your heart.

Sun Pose

Sun Pose is really a gesture of glowing pleasure that obviously deepens the breath.

Do: Raise your arms overhead, then stretch your hands and Fingers, and softly appear.

Feel: The duration and raise of your upper body along with The movement of breath on your stomach and rib cage.

The Yoga Warrior

The warrior poses strengthen the Entire Body when Assisting You link to inner peace and strength.

Start into: Peaceful warrior pose

Inhale: Courageous Warrior pose

Exhale: Peaceful Warrior pose

Peaceful Warrior Pose

Peaceful warrior has an Chance to practice Lounging to breathe and feeling, without needing to do anything or change anything.

Do: Stand with one foot forward of the Other and much apart to develop to a cosy gliding (for brave warrior). Examine this by bending your knee. Ensure the front knee ceases directly on the front head, perhaps not all of the way across the feet. Then relax back to a resting posture, both arms with your palms in your own heart. Close your lips or eyes in your palms.

Feel: The power and steadiness of all Your thighs, the relaxation of your own face, and also the motion of breath wherever your hands combine your heart.

Courageous Warrior Pose

Courageous warrior brings power to the whole body and

is a chance to relate to the sense of fulfilling life with a open heart and willing spirit.

Do: Bend front knee and raise your arms overhead, so maintaining The neck and shoulders relaxed. Gradually appear. Since you extend your arms and palms upward, ground down throughout the toes like rooting to the ground.

Feel: The devotion of the legs, powerful and rested; the motion of the breath on your stomach, ribs, and torso; and also a Feeling of this Entire body glowing with energy.

Strength and Surrender

This Sequence strengthens and Moves the Entire Body while researching two very different methods of fulfilling a question: dedication and letting go.

Start in: Mountain pose

Inhale: Fierce Pose

Exhale: Forward fold

Optional Step: Return pose following every cycle to break For a single breath.

Fierce pose

Fierce pose strengthens the Entire body and Heart and Provides a chance to practice reassurance and steadiness at a challenging circumstance.

Do: Bend your knees, then sit hips Back, and then lean the chest forward. Lift your arms and keep the spine as quickly as you can. Don't forget to breathe.

Feel: Notice the senses of Work In this particular pose, which can be very hard to hold. Be curious about the way the senses of work and strength change in the senses of fatigue and pain. Can you remain in this pose with both stamina and devotion but not intense distress?

Forward fold

Forward fold releases pressure from the Arms, neck, shoulders, back, buttocks, and thighs, and has been an chance to practice letting go of unneeded bodily or psychological stress.

Do: Using slightly flexed legs fold Forward in the hips. Relax your spine and upper body and then allow gravity pull you to the pose. It isn't important how much you move, provided that you're relaxational.

Feel: The feeling of stretch on your back, buttocks, and thighs along with the feeling of relaxed heaviness on your upper torso. How Is it true that the feeling of elongate differ in the pain? Can you unwind to the Feeling and keep in this pose without even performing anything except letting go?

Bowing in Gratitude

This sequence carries just two of the Ideal Full-body moves in most yoga and joins them together to express reverence and gratitude for every single breath and every moment.

This flowUtilizes a new Breathing pattern which slows down the transition between poses. Always proceed between both poses on the inhalation and then hold each pose for a single exhalation.

Inhale: Start on hands and knees

Exhale: Proceed to next posture (downward-facing dog pose or Kid's pose)

Downward-facing dog

Downward-facing dog releases pressure from the legs, chest, shoulders, and spine while developing strength at the upper body.

Do: By an all-fours place, lift Your knees and start to lift your buttocks. Press down on the palms and draw on your shoulders and hips up and back. Gradually straighten your legs to grow the stretch, or maintain your knees flexed if that is much more relaxational.

Feel: The link of the palms to the floor and the feeling of power at the upper body; the link of the toes into the floor and the feeling of stretch at the body; the stream of breath in and from the nose, mouth, and neck.

Child pose

Child pose releases stress From the buttocks, shoulders, back, and torso and is a complete - figure gesture of confidence in, and gratitude to get the current moment.

Do: Drop to your knees, then draw your buttocks Rear toward the heels, then break your belly onto the thighs, and then break your arms and head onto the floor. If your buttocks can't touch with your heels, or your knees are somewhat uneasy as you can hold this pose, put a blanket or pillow between the heels and hips.

Feel: The motion of breath at the Stomach and spine, and also a feeling of gratitude on your thoughts and heart.

Cobra Rising

This Sequence powerfully Reinforces the back of Your System and Educates you how To keep a balance of work and simplicity.

Start: Constructed on tummy

Inhale: Cobra pose

Exhale: Resting cobra

Cobra Pose

This pose strengthens the legs and back and Embodies the capacity to rise above adversity.

Do: Bring your arms from the side, Either bent together with your hands from the torso or stretched back along with your buttocks. When you inhale, lift your headback, chest, shoulders, and thighs. Come only as much as you're able to keep a relaxational breath. After holding the pose, remain in 50 to 60 percent max attempt and enable the elevation of this pose to naturally grow and drop somewhat because you breathe.

Feel: The potency of your body, The willingness of your torso as you inhale, and also the subtle increase and collapse in the upper body as you breathe.

Resting cobra

This pose is a Chance to practice resting And receiving aid when attempt is no more desired.

Do: Relax in your own belly. Create a comfy resting Location to your arms and mind.

Feel: The help of the floor underneath you and The motion of the breath on your stomach and back again.

The Drawbridge

The Drawbridge strengthens and moves the whole body.

Start: working on your back, with legs bent and feet on the floor, knees and toes hips-distance aside

Inhale: Bridge pose

Exhale: Knees-to-chest pose

Bridge pose

Bridge pose assembles Strength from the thighs, buttocks, and heart and releases tension from the shoulders and torso.

Do: In one easy motion, lift your arms toward the ground and then reduced them into the ground behind you, since you push down through your heels lift your buttocks and lower back off the floor. Keep your knees straight on your toes, not slipping out into either side or grinding together.

Feel: The link of your toes to the floor, the power of your thighs, and also the motion of the breath on your stomach, rib cage, and torso.

Knees-to-chest

Knees-to-chest Pose releases tension from the back and hips.

Do: Hug your knees in your stomach and chest. Keep your mind and shoulders Relaxed on the floor.

Feel: The help of the floor underneath you and The motion of the stomach from the thighs as you inhale.

Sweet Dreams

This Sequence is created of three-sided poses. It's a lullaby for your human body and a great transition in the final relaxation pose. It's possible to practice every pose on either side of your system before continuing on to another pose or exercise each of three poses on a single side of your system prior to switching sides and beginning the sequence above. This sequence works well as a slow stream, holding each pose for five to ten breaths prior to going into another pose.

Cradle Pose

Cradle Pose releases tension from the buttocks, buttocks, and spine.

Do: Cross one foot on the other leg close to the knee. Draw the base leg toward your stomach and clasp your hands on the other side of the thigh or throughout the groove. Keep your head and shoulders rested on the floor.

Feel: The feeling of stretch on your Outer hip and inner thigh, the heaviness of the shoulders and head resting on the ground, and also the rise and fall of your stomach as you breathe.

Resting twist

Resting twist releases pressure from the abdomen, torso, Shoulders, shoulders, and hips and obviously deepens the breath.

Do: Start with knees on your own Stomach and drop both arms to one side. Stretch out your arms to both sides. Don't push your thighs, shoulders, arms or arms into the floor whenever they don't inherently touch. Relax and allow gravity pull you to the pose. You may always put a blanket or cushion beneath any part of the human body that doesn't touch the floor.

Feel: The Feeling of gravity attracting you To the pose, the help of the floor under you, as well as also the inhalation stretching the abdomen and chest from the interior.

Half Moon Pose

Half-moon pose releases tension across the entire Side of their human body and can be an chance to exercise doing less to get more.

Do: Start lying on your back. Walk equally heels to a side until you feel A stretch from the cervical or cool. Cross one ankle on the opposite. Press down your elbows to lift the shoulders and then transfer them in exactly the exact same way as your own heels. Relax your arms on the floor overhead and pull gently to the stretch. Keep toes, shoulders, buttocks, and arms onto the floor.

Feel: The senses of stretch across both sides of thighs, hips, chest, waist, and shoulders; also the link with your heels, hips, chest, head, and hands inside out; the inhalation stretching the belly and chest from the inside out.

RELAXATION CAN RELIEVE YOUR PAIN

Relaxation sounds like the simplest thing on the planet till you attempt to unwind, and all a sudden, it is hopeless. You provide the control to unwind, but your body and mind could be stubborn in lots of ways! From racing ideas to muscles which refuse to go, what is assumed to become blissful could become stressful. When you're in pain, lying down and shutting your eyes could be downright terrifying since you wind up having nothing to do however feel and consider your pain.

Whether this description of relaxation has you believing it may be a fantastic idea to jump to another chapter, continue. Total relaxation of body and mind is possible also yes, as dreadful as its guarantee. It's, in actuality, the perfect treatment for both chronic strain and pain. This chapter will instruct you step-by-step to unwind with 2 yoga relaxation methods, mindful relaxation and healing yoga.

Why is relaxation so valuable for chronic pain? To start out with, relaxation is instantly curing. It ends the pressure reaction and arouses the human body's energy to increase, repair, immune function, digestion, and additional self-nurturing procedures. Doctor Herbert Benson called this therapeutic manner the"relaxation response".

Relaxation also functions within the long run to make a clean slate to your body and mind. The relaxation response tightens the mind-body samskaras, which bring about pain and offers the basis for curing customs. Consistent relaxationpractice instructs the body and mind the way to break in a feeling of security instead of chronic emergency. After the human body and mind feel secure, it's a lot easier to direct them toward the adventure of profound inner peace and joy.

Would you unwind as you're in pain? Yes. It is not just possible; it ought to grow into one of the very first approaches when you locate your pain becoming worse. Pain is precisely the opportunity to try out a relaxation practice, even when encounter isn't as blissful as relaxation whenever you aren't in distress. Provided that the position you're in isn't creating your pain worse, then provide relaxationa opportunity to show its advantages to you. Relaxation can operate in mysterious ways, such as providing you with a better feeling of control over the pain and guts to take care of your pain.

Relaxation also trains your body and mind to distinguish the senses of bodily pain in the full-out crisis response. That is the reason why relaxation helps if it does not eliminate all your pain. If it's possible to relax even if you're in physical pain, then you also can untangle the knots on your nervous system which link all kinds of distress and pain. Many individuals with chronic pain discover that pain mechanically triggers a stress reaction, and stress mechanically worsens pain. If the clot joining physical pain and stress are all untangled, you can break this cycle. The body and mind learn to possess more nuanced responses to life's struggles. If it's possible to learn how to relax while in pain, then you'll realize that pain and stress are no more the mind-body's automatic reaction to every challenging moment.

Conscious Relaxation

Consciously stressed and relax the entire body, 1 place at one time. Rush between regions. **Exercise:**

Lyingright down, or at any other place if lying is unrelaxationable.To release tension and tension within your system.

During stress or pain, episodes to change attention and

also to find a Feeling of Security, management, and relaxation.

In mattress Before sleeping to help conquer insomnia linked to stress or pain.

A full-body practice takes five to ten minutes.

Let us Try out a small experimentation in relaxation: lift your shoulders as large as possible on your ears. Squeeze these tight! Let head, and allow the shoulders fall. Try so again, only now with all the breath: inhale as you lift your shoulders as large as possible, and exhale through your mouth because you shed them. Now, take action, just raise your shoulders as large, using just half the hard work and strain. Try this one more time, without much less effort, raising the shoulders just a little. Exhale, and go entirely.

The following step requires Shutting your eyes. You are likely to repeat the entire procedure, but on your own imagination only. With your eyes shut, picture lifting your shoulders as large as possible to your own ears because you inhale and falling them because you exhale. Try this a couple times, picturing stress and then imagining relaxation. Envision whole attempt, then half attempt, then half an attempt. Then break your shoulders and then notice your breathagain. Keep your eyes shut and require a couple of moments to just see the way you're feeling.

So, how can it go? Are you currently really able to tense your shoulders purpose? If this is so, you've taken a significant first step in figuring out how to unwind. Allergic pressure can appear as a step in the wrong way, but it could really help purify the entire human body and head for relaxation.

Here is why: the majority of the strain that you hold on your own body is unconscious and unintentional. This is 1-way chronic pain may creep up on you--unconscious habits of stress fly beneath the radar till suddenly the stress turns into annoyance. The issue isthat you can not let go of stress you are not mindful of and are not performing on goal.

The yoga exercise of Conscious relaxation follows the principle it is simpler to reverse something you're doing on goal than something you're doing . During conscious relaxation, you may stressed distinct regions of your body on function and then give up that attempt. Just because you did with your own shoulders at the relaxation experimentation, you may begin with large movement and work your way to much more subtle pressure and release. The rounds which use just your creative work in a deeper degree of retraining the body and mind. Imagery functions on unconscious tension, permitting this around to dissolve stress you can't control at will.

Through time, You'll discover that a normal practice of mindful relaxation makes it simpler to fall in the healing condition of the complete relaxation reaction. You'll also gain increased awareness of where and when you hold tension in the human entire body. With this knowledge and the ability of conscious relaxation, you'll have the ability to give up that strain at will.

Conscious relaxation May be practised at any position which you find comfy, such as seated, standing, or bending down.

Begin with a place of Your body which you truly feel as though you have more conscious control over. This probably Won't be some area of your body where you hold experience or strain pain. Work your way into people Chronically stressed and painful places as soon as you've established relaxation in Other regions of the human body. If you've A record of muscular aches or accidents in a place, forget the very first step of this Procedure (full strain) and begin with a few of those gentle variations, either utilizing Less effort or beginning with the creativity around.

Follow the tips below to any or all these areas of the body:

Hands and wrists

Arms

Neck and shoulders

Confront

Torso

Stomach

Back

Buttocks

Legs

Ankles and feet

Creating Tension And Letting Go

There Are Several Ways to Stressed a body area. Do not fret about if you're doing this exactly the correct way. From the very first round, make the type of stress that moves the part of the body you're working with. Squeezelift, lift, tighten, contract, and pull, and push--anything makes sense for this body area. To go ahead, just quit doing the energetic strain. The outcome will undoubtedly be relaxation. Repeat the motion a couple of occasions, but with increasingly less attempt to strain every moment.

From the creativity rounds, Shut your eyes and picture the activities you performed. Imagine the sensation of this strain and release. You could realize that imagining jelqing and letting go proceeds to release stress, despite the fact that you're not actively pursuing the muscle . That is normal and a fantastic indication that the procedure is functioning. In case the creativity round feels confusing or hard, you can make it all out. You might find it simpler, initially, to operate with just the huge tense-and-release around, since this may be a lot easier to control. In cases like this, you may add the creativity around in after sessions.

Breathing

You will notice that occasionally It's easier to Create stress if you inhale (by way of instance, the back or shoulder) and occasionally it's a lot easier to make strain

If You exhale (by way of instance, the stomach or buttocks). The absolute most significant issue is to earn the breath part of the procedure. Experiment with your breathing to determine which regions stressed more obviously within the exhalation and then tense more obviously on the inhalation. Provided that you aren't holding the breath, anything routine you follow would be just nice. Make sure you rest at a relaxed breath between both rounds of tensing and releasing your body.

Resting

Between body regions, Pause for a few breaths and then notice how you're feeling. To highlight the ramifications of conscious relaxation, you may use the Development of firming the entire Body for every region of the body once you consciously stressed and unwind it. Imagine inhaling and exhaling out of every part of the human body, and envision any lingering strain being dissolved from the breath. You might even utilize a light/colour visualization through the resting period. Once you consciously stressed and launch a place of the human body, shut your eyes and envision that region gently glowing with a shade you associate with recovery, relaxation, and relaxation. From the time that you are completed with the whole practice, you can envision the entire body glowing with mild or your recovery colour.

Restorative yoga

Restorative yoga ends up on the recovery Relaxation answer by blending gentle yoga poses together with mindful meditation and breathing. In the subsequent pages, you'll find five restorative yoga poses which could possibly be practised by themselves or inside a sequence.

There are a couple of things That produce restorative yoga really calming. To begin with, every pose is supposed to be kept for more than a couple breaths. You are able to remain in a therapeutic posture for ten minutes or more. The stillness makes it possible for the entire body to fall even the deepest levels of stress.

Secondly, restorative Poses utilize props to back up your

physique. Props may incorporate the walls, a chair, a sofa, cushions, towels, blankets, or bolsters made particularly for restorative yoga training. The ideal support at a pose can make it feel simple, which means that your body is able to completely let go.

You Also should not feel powerful sensations of strength or stretch how that you are at a more lively yoga pose. Stretching and strengthening, though

Healthful, are both kinds of stress from the entire body. They're a type of very good strain on your system, asking the human body to adapt to the struggles of a particular pose. Restorative yoga is about letting go of stress and stress. You may adapt the poses to your entire body, with whatever props create your body feel fantastic just because it is. Since you hold each pose, start looking for a grade of simplicity within the human body and the breath that appears mild or even impartial.

Ultimately, though these poses might look like You're doing nothing, this can be not anywhere near the reality. Restorative Yoga rests your human body but engages the brain. The meditation and breathing parts Of every pose create restorative yoga an energetic process of concentrating the mind on recovery ideas, Sensations, and feelings.

YOGA STRATEGIES FOR LASTING NECK RELIEF

I believe you've Realize how yoga Can enable one to alleviate and eliminate pain in your shoulders and neck. And I expect it is also apparent that yoga isn't only a workout but in addition a detailed approach to self-indulgent and transformation which involves many different practices done either on and off the yoga mat. While the tradition of yoga poses is very essential to boost the strength, versatility, and appropriate hygiene essential to removing shoulder and neck pain, the easy practice of consciousness during your day may also have a profound impact. Meditation asks us to look closely at the many facets which could influence shoulder and neck pain--such as postural habits, body mechanics, ideas, and feelings --and also proceed with compassion and diligence from the path of wellbeing.

And unlike other Therapeutic choices --for example, visiting a physician, nurse, or acupuncturist--yoga is something which just you may perform to your self . While a seasoned yoga teacher or yoga therapist might help lead you with this interior battle of self-discovery and self-indulgent, the practice will be grounded on your very own personal explorations and opinions --and your own relationship with your "inner teacher" Yoga isn't a"one size fits all" job. It is a personalized exercise, tailored to match your distinctive structure, history, character, character, and requirements. Plus it takes one to take responsibility to your own aftercare, a strategy currently recognized by Western health specialists as critically important for individuals with neck pain.

As a complement to this More detailed directions posted in the remainder of this book, I provide this Concise overview of eight fundamental self-care strategies for healthier neck and shoulders:

On the mat

 1. Regular Yoga Exercise: Produce a dedication to

performing a few formal yoga training daily. By proper, I do not indicate you need to always wear a particular outfit or invest a lot of time. (See chapter 5 to certain recommendations how long, where, and when to practice) However, It's

Essentialtomake your yoga training a Daily habit , even for a brief time every day, you cease all of the busyness of accomplishing, preparation, and trying so you're able to turn your focus inward, be pose within your own body and breathe, stretch, relax, and energize. While, ideally, this will occur onto a yoga mat, conditions might necessitate your practice happen elsewhere, maybe in a hotel area, on your workplace, or at bed. My instructor, Esther Myers, who died of cancer in January 2004, after explained that until she had cancer, then she believed yoga postures completed in bed did not count, which you needed to do the bearings on the ground in order for it to be Pilates. But following her cancer diagnosis, she understood that it is about yoga.

Off or on the mat

2. Breathing Practice: Slow, deep breathing is character's Own anti-stress medication, and it is Free, easy, and right beneath your nose. Breathing is the sole bodily function which you may do either consciously or unconsciously, and that is controlled by two distinct forms of nerves and joints: involuntary and voluntary. If you have conscious charge of your breath, then it opens the door to relaxing with your nervous system. Or, since yoga pro B. K. S. Iyengar describes in his classic manual, Light on Yoga,"permeates the breathing, and thus restrain the brain" (Iyengar 1979, 21).

So take some time Daily to concentrate on your breath. This is sometimes a part of your formal practice to the mat or even something that you informally weave in your daily life, by way of instance, while waiting in a traffic light or in a physician's office, or in case you are feeling stress. A number of the students tell me that they utilize breathing practice to assist them fall asleep during night or maybe to return to sleep whenever they awaken during the evening time.

Particular instructions on deep abdominal breathing are all provided In phase 5. To Enhance your expertise, try Both of These fundamental breathing techniques:

Even Breath: Switch your focus to a breath, also emotionally count The period of your inhalation and also the period of your exhalation. Then attempt to produce your inhalation and exhalation equivalent length. By way of instance, you might count"one, two, three, four" in your own inhalation and"one, two, three, four" in your exhalation. Or you might rely on five, five, or even six; it does not matter. Simply do your very best to create your inhalation and exhalation precisely the identical length. Proceed for three to four minutes, then let your breath return to its natural rhythm.

Extended Exhalation: Start using the breath (previously); subsequently perform Producing your exhalation around two as long as the inhalation. As an instance, if you inhale to the count of four, then consider exhaling to the count of five, seven, six, or even eight. Much like yoga training, prevent strain. Simply do your very best to create your exhalation more in the inhalation. This is sometimes an especially relaxing practice.

3. Meditation: When you have ever seen a gorgeous

sunset, stared in a candle flame, or gazed in a persuasive picture or statue, then you have practised meditation. Regardless of the frequent misperception that meditation demands draining the brain, meditation really entails filling your brain with an item of attention, make it a fire, film, blossom, deity, colour, audio, or almost anything. Meditation is just one of yoga's most important parts, as both the religious practice and a highly effective healing methodology. Considering that the meditator repeats integration, becoming one with the object of attention, it is helpful to select as the object of meditation that which that you find attractive that is also constructive, effective, and recovery, like an inspirational phrase or prayer. "The important thing is altering the brain in a favourable manner," yoga pro-T. K. V. Desikachar explained when I interviewed him for an article in Yoga Journal,"since anything happens in the brain occurs in the entire method" (Krucoff 2007).

Among my favourite meditations would be the next:

Mantra Meditation: A mantra is merely a thought or goal expressed as a noise that is employed as an outcome of meditation. For Your headline, select a phrase, a word, Or a line of a prayer or poem that is significant to you. An example May Be that the Dorothy headline: There is no place like home. Recite this mantra, either quietly or Out loud, once in your inhalation and after on Your own exhalation. Or, to get a version of this extended Exhalation practice over, Recite it on inhalation and double on exhalation. To start, place a Timer for 3 minutes and attempt to remain focused on your own headline the entire moment. When other thoughts appear, detect without ruling Your head is chattering Then return your attention to your own headline. As time passes, you may try increasing the period of time spent meditating.

Off-The-Mat Practices

4. Incorporate Yoga to Daily Life: Fundamentally, this implies listen to what is happening with yourself emotionally, emotionally, mentally, and emotionally during daily.

Do your best to:

- Sit, Stand, and proceed with great posture.
- Prevent Staying at a predetermined position for long; awaken and stretchand walk a little, breathe.
- Weave short yoga"micro-practices" in daily. For Instance, Do some basic postures in your desk (for instance, shoulder shrugs, squeeze arms(and seated rear bend) or if you are standing online (for instance, mountain posture, tree pose(and also mild twist). Get in the practice of carrying a complete, deep breath until you answer your phone. Use waiting period at a red light or if the computer boots upas an chance to perform a meditation.
- Regularly bring your consciousness into your neck and neck; maybe put your alarm to ring each hour, and see if you are holding pressure in this region (such as your own mouth, face, arms, and upper spine). If this is so, have a deep breath, and then encourage your own muscles to relax and discharge.

5. Develop a Supportive Environment: Ensure that your physical environment support healthful posture--in the office, in your vehicle, and in your home. Get the gear you want to keep your shoulders and neck in good posture, like a phone headset, along with a correctly fitted seat and computer desk with accessories that are necessary, such as, for instance, a file holder. Attempt to maintain your lively surroundings healthy by reducing clutter and clutter. Cultivate a supportive social environment by strengthening positive connections with people that you care about and also nourishing excellent friendships. If you realize your shoulders and neck become stressed once you're about a specific individual, avoid spending some time with this particular individual or work on enhancing the connection.

6. Self-Study: Among those self-discipline practices (niyamas) summarized at the Yoga Sutras of Patanjali is svadhyaya, meaning"study" This practice identifies to research of texts and self-study, and it is a car for self-understanding and, in the end, transformation. Among the most effective strategies to find out more about your self -- your own habits, ideas, and feelings -- would be to maintain a journal or a practice that is often suggested for people managing chronic pain. Look at keeping tabs on your own pain level from daily, maybe utilizing a 0 to 10 scale, where 0 is"no-hassle" and 10 is"the worst pain possible" Specifically, notice exactly what you've already been performing (physically, mentally, and emotionally) on times when you are experiencing elevated levels of shoulder and neck pain, and see whether you're able to tease out the causes associated with greater pain. Additionally, you might choose to write about stressful events and document your own ideas and feelings. The initial act of reposing in your own life and writing down everything you think and believe could be curative. Writing in a diary may help you shed light on factors which give rise to your neck disrelaxation, find out on your patterns of behaviour and thought, and supply options for recovery.

7. Self-Care Tool Kit: Particular tools could be useful in helping alleviate pain, such as:

Body tools: Exercise balls, foam rollers, the Thera Cane, along with other body parts may Help you get especially tight muscles and supply help in helping discharge tension. Look at utilizing these tools along with breathing exercise, encouraging your muscles to discharge with every exhalation. (See the resources section for advice about places to purchase body resources.)

Ice packs: I usually maintain a couple of tender ice packs Inside my freezer (available at most drugstores) for emergency first aid, because ice may be secure and beneficial approach to reduce inflammation and alleviate pain. You might even use a bag of frozen corn or peas, which moulds well around curved body parts such as the shoulders and neck. Make certain to put a towel between your skin and the ice hockey. Individuals are frequently confused as to when to utilize ice hockey and when to use heat for pain relief. The general guideline is ice to get a brand new or severe pain and warmth for an older or chronic pain. But if it is a pain that has been around for a little while, if you are using a flare-up, ice might be a fantastic option. Experiment and find out which one works best.

Heat pads and hot bathrooms: To soothe persistent stiffness and aches, think about applying Warmth using a heating system or soaking in a hot tub. To help alleviate muscular aches, include Epsom salts and essential oils into the bath, employing a relaxing odour like lavender or lavender.

8. Set up a support Team: Construct a community of caregivers that will help you fulfil your objectives. Based upon your personal situation and requirements, your system could contain doctors, massage therapists, acupuncturists, physical therapists, therapists, psychotherapists, yoga therapists, and yoga instructors. But try to remember that you're responsible for your health; see these professionals since your advisers and partners that provide you with their knowledge and assist you in making the best decisions for your personal recovery. Think about attending to a regular yoga course, directed by an experienced and respectful teacher (see the tools section for assistance locating one). Being a part of a community of like-mindedd seekers, also called sangha, maybe a really sterile experience. However, ensure your yoga course is a match to your normal home practice, maybe not a replacement for this.

These self-care Approaches aren't "commandments"; they're not carved in rock! They are simply ideas for measures you may take to exploit the healing power of yoga. As always, use what works for you and dismiss the remainder.

And Keep in Mind, be Thankful that you possess a neck and Shoulders even if they are painful. Be kind to them, so listen to these, and do your best to take the necessary Actions to cultivate Recovery within this difficult region --and within your complete body, mind, and soul. Let every inhalation be an Chance to Satisfy your being with recovery energy. And allow every exhalation be a Opportunity To unwind, discharge, and let go of pain, nervousness, And whatever else you do not require.

CHAPTER FIVE

❦

YOGA RITUAL

Making Your Own Morning Yoga Ritual

The next ideas can help you develop with your yoga ritual to practice daily.

Linking to your Body and breath will provide you more energy and excitement to deal with daily. Pick your favourite breathing workout and follow along using a few of your favourite two-pose escapes.

Shamatha (befriending The mind) is the ideal meditation practise for the first thing in the afternoon. The clarity and attention you grow will take in the remainder of the day, assisting you to make conscious decisions that support your health and wellbeing.

CittaBhavana Meditations are a superb means to establish your goal for your day. What you decide to concentrate on initial thing may affect how you have the remainder of your daily life. Which of those meditations appealed to you personally? Pick among these meditations and also make it the morning ritual, either in or out of bed.

Take 1 thing that you do each morning, shower, make coffee, cook and insert your favourite headline Meditation for it.

Making Your Own Evening Yoga Rituals

These ideas might inspire your evening yoga ritual.

Relaxation helps to Unravel the strain of this day and prepare one to get a fantastic night's sleep. Pick at least one of your treasured restorative yoga poses and also include any breathing or meditation practice that provides you peace of mind.

The day is an Fantastic time to irritate your physique. Which of those expressions or meditations within prior chapters appealed the most to youpersonally? Create a ritual of hammering about these expressions, or practising these meditations, every evening.

Lots of yoga Practices may be completed in bed, and several will make it a lot easier to fall asleep. A number of the very best pre-sleep practices would be the aid breath, and breathing the entire body, conscious relaxation, mantra meditation, cittaBhavana meditations, as well as the pratipakshaBhavana meditation finding opposites within the entire body.

Here are some other questions That Will Help You locate your Yoga rituals:

Why Can you opt to start a yoga practice? What's the intention to your practice? Of all of the practices, you have heard in this novel, which helps the best or most reflects this aim?

Of The practices, you have attempted in every phase, which supplies you with the best feeling of confidence? Which supplies you with the best feeling of energy? Try some of those practices, or set them collectively, as a ritual.

Which Of the practices within this book supplies you with the best feeling of relaxation and calmness? Which supplies you with the best relief from stress or stress? Try out these practices within a day ritual.

What Practice provides you the best sense of linking to your internal wisdom--the capability to become a guide on your head, listen to your own body, and pick an adventure of peace? Try out this practice for a morning or night ritual.

What Practice provides you the best feeling of linking to a normal pleasure --the feeling of gratitude, openness to confront life, and also being linked to something larger? Try out this practice for a morning or night ritual.

CentreYourself with a couple of minutes of relaxation, breath awareness, or meditation. Then ask yourself, "What's my yoga ?" Trust your inner knowledge.

You Might Find it Helpful to document your morning and night rituals. If You Prefer, you can utilize The subsequent blank pages to spell out your personal rituals.

HATHA YOGA

Considering that the mid-20th century, hatha yoga has become a very popular alternative for men and women that wish to boost their thoughts, body and health. This early practice is intended to promote balance between these 3 elements. In reality, the term "yoga" really refers to the marriage, literally the "yoking together" of religious, physical and psychological wellness. Hatha yoga gives a balanced, recovery approach to release stress, improve physical illness, and increase relaxation for people around the world.

This kind of yoga is thought to be one of the significant kinds of yoga training, together with kundalini yoga, karma yoga and several more. It's the parent of many different sorts of yoga, like Bikram yoga, which employs a similar sequence but adds additional challenges like a very hot area. All yoga exercise originates from religious areas that began around 5,000 decades past, though these actions weren't exactly the same as the current hatha yoga. Ancient meditative and bodily practices finally evolved into a kind that contemporary professionals would recognize.

They stayed a relatively unknown procedure of personal progress until the 1960s and 1970s, but when considering oriental practices improved greatly. The development of interest in other treatments led more individuals in Europe and North America to embrace and adapt yogic practices for their use, making the yoga courses we currently see as standard.

The course slowly develops tougher, but a lot of them offer alternate variations of these poses, or asanas, to permit disabled people or people in poor physical condition to take part. Some versions, such as ashtanga yoga, are very busy, while conventional Hatha practice is comparatively slow. The following session of meditation completes the course, enabling participants to"cool down."

Ways to Benefit from Hatha Yoga

Scientific studies have revealed that routine hatha yoga practice delivers lots of physical and psychological advantages. For example, those who have eating disorders experienced fitter relationships with meals after they practised yoga compared to once they didn't. This historical art can create substantial stress, depression and stress relief, also. It promotes mindfulness and makes it simpler to take even quite difficult events peacefully and without intense distress.

Hatha yoga professionals are demonstrated to have greater flexibility, posture and coordination compared to those who do not engage in this kind of exercise. Patients with medical issues can do better with yoga, also. While there is no evidence that yoga can cure cardiovascular disease, cancer or other serious ailments, it may have significant positive outcomes.

HATHA YOGA BENEFITS

The chief objective of Hatha Yoga is substantially the same as different kinds of yoga training. It tries to combine the soul of the person with the increased soul of the world, enhancing the health of the soul, mind, emotions and body. Hatha Yoga was said to assist professionals attain inner peace and a sense of oneness with the world. Bear in mind that regardless of which kind of yoga you decide to do, immersion is a really significant element.

All sorts of yoga have a few similarities. But they differ in purpose or methods in different regions. Hatha Yoga's most important focus is the preparation of their human body so the soul will have the ability to do its role in bringing the professional to enlightenment. A lot of confusion may arise, as a lot of folks don't recognize it is important to get a healthy, healthy body so as to successfully achieve spiritual enlightenment.

Hatha Yoga practice is placed on the entire body so as to

fortify it and the soul inside. Its bodily techniques are frequently employed by those that aren't interested in spiritual improvement, but who'd love to get the physical advantages of Hatha Yoga also.

Along with the physical advantages of Hatha Yoga, in addition, there are mental ones. It has been stated to help in the evolution of higher focusing and concentration skills, besides reducing tension and stress. For a lot of , this can be a significant advantage and something that they want in their own lives. If you are being diverted and want a while to unwind, Hatha Yoga may be the ideal alternative.

For people that are trying to find a spiritual advantage, Hatha Yoga permits you to discover your very own heavenly light. Additionally, it can help you become more powerful, more elastic, and much more relaxed. Performing Hatha Yoga enables the power of your soul to flow freely because the brain, soul, and body are more tightly at harmony. Sceptical? Consider how difficult it's to focus when you've got a headache.

Practising Hatha Yoga will help you deal with stress, and can alleviate some of your pain and nervousness. When work is leaving you tired, you have to find time to unwind and renew yourself. Hatha Yoga is a great remedy, which will be able to enable you to release built-up anxieties and stress.

BHAKTI YOGA

Bhakti Yoga is much more of a religious idea of the practice of Yoga. Although many Yoga methods orient themselves in the bodily and psychological advances, Bhakti focuses primarily on the religious connection between the person and God.

The foundation of Bhakti can be summed up as a series. This series begins at the base of God, Himself, goes through all facts and finishes in the core of the person. This series is always powerful at the stage of Gods' toes since God is omniscient rather than changing. On the people ending, however, life may wear in the series, weakening it. The person, through Bhakti Yoga, altered the essence of the series, making it new life and power. The result is that of a more powerful religious connection with the Maker.

By means of this early form of Yogawe arrive at the understanding that God's love is the purest type of love potential, not hurtful, not misleading, never neglecting, rather than under any conditions, vindictive at all. It's the best love. Bhakti instructs us that man may attain this love since man is made in the image of God. It's very simple to deduce that, with all these facts in your mind, person can understand through Bhakti, to adore God as He loves uspurely and unselfishly.

The true term, Bhakti, arises in the term Bhaj, that translates neatly to'attachment to God.' In the true practice of the particular format of Yoga, there are numerous quite powerful and desired sockets, for example,Sakamya, Nishkamya, Japa, and Upasana, to list a couple.

Sakarya is most likely the least preferred, in it is a self-centred kind of Bhakti. Sakamya is a pursuit, through Bhakti, to attain increased substance gains here in the world, and more oriented towards the gratifying of and connection with God. Japa is additionally a self-centred kind of Bhakti, however not too much for substance needs but for bodily demands. By way of instance, if a person suffers from cancer and needs God to cure him, he plays a daily ritual of Japa Bhakti Yoga.

The fundamental principles of Bhakti are that if you're truly in your mind and will willingly experience the procedure of Bhakti to reach them, then God will give your orders as he's promised. Nevertheless, with no good carved in rock ethical outlook, to do Bhakti is moot.

JUANA YOGA

You might have heard Jnana Yoga is "Union via comprehension," but most Yoga pupils continue to be profoundly saddened by this explanation. The deeper explanation for Jnana Yoga is lengthy and complicated. Jnana is a religious discipline, which allows you to start the instinctive powers of your spirit. The analysis of Jnana Yoga has been full of self-inquiry along with self-discovery.

The consequence of this pursuit is understanding of this Supreme Being that we call God, Brahman, Allah, Yahweh, Jehovah, The Total, and a lot more titles. The assortment of titles for the Supreme Being unimportant.

Every one of us sees, feels, hears, smells, and tastes, and whatever otherwise. 1 man enjoys the flavour of something, while the other doesn't. If you like something and somebody else doesn't, in the event you ever judge them harshly or think an enemy to them? This frequently occurs in politics, sports, faith, as well as driving through traffic.

People must get beyond their differences to be able find their authentic and greater goal in life. Critically estimating each other, and ourselves absorbs a great deal of energy in the kind of anger, stress, stress, jealousy, and hate.

Regrettably, some individuals won't ever get beyond their differences, unless they genuinely need to modify. World peace are the final result of international Jnana Yoga practice. Realization of God makes us conscious of the place in the world.

Jnana Yoga is a self-quest, a travel inside, self-realization, and transformation, and all wrapped into a single package. Study, Pranayama, meditation, and Japa are still Only a few those elements inside Jnana Yoga.

Throughout the class of Jnana Yoga research, the practitioner learns to determine their authentic self, and what we call the"witness" The opinion isn't a judge, but not your own character, rather than your ideas. The watch is the impartial observer of all of the right and wrong you've done daily.

Still, the witness may take care of each these items and forgive you on your own shortcomings. The watch doesn't own a good deal of "hang-ups." The watch has ever been celebrating that the "monkey brain" inside each people. The watch doesn't laugh , because the watch is much removed from the ego.

So, how can we get in contact with the remark? How do we provide this impartial observer a bit more power in crucial circumstances? The majority of us want a non-judging watch to assist us with starvation, anger, stress, stress, jealousy, and despise daily. This opinion would earn a fantastically.

Primarily we will need to really look in the mirror. What

do people find? Can we position ourselves? How long do people spend daily, encouraging our egos? Just how many judgment calls are all influenced by our past social conditioning?

The responses to the majority of our issues are inside us. The authentic ego is like an onion, using tough outer layers of character, which the entire world sees. These outer layers constitute our mask. We need to be cautious that the outer layers of conditioning and self aren't in complete control.

The outer layers of character carry arbitrary idea and don't necessarily make the best choices, but they really do believe your own self-protection first. Random ideas and self-realization are substantially different.

Which of those two would you want to deal with a disaster situation? The self-realized head has integrity and isn't in a hurry to generate rash decisions or even harsh conclusions. This is the end result of Jnana Yoga practice.

Jnana Yoga is frequently known as "marriage by understanding." Jnana can be called, "the course of wisdom" A Jnana Yoga pro dedicates much time ahead of training, study, and self-analysis. Traditionally, this procedure of Yoga has been practised by most members of their Brahman (priest) caste.

The cause of this was predicated upon a necessity of instruction and basic understanding. If a person has limited skills to see, then chief education has to be achieved first. Add to this, the sort of reading that you has to play - the sorting and absorption of facts out of scriptures and instructional books with dependable details.

To read dependable advice is to enlarge the brain in a

favourable direction. To read misinformation direct you to "spout off" truth, that can not exist. Have you ever noticed somebody create a incorrect announcement, based on an"urban legend" Posts? Nearly all of the material is governmental; however, misinformation occurs in Yoga circles also.

We live at a period when lots of individuals have access to the world wide web. However, just how much of this info online is true? It may be smart to double-check your details before investing too much time in them. There are individuals who purchase magazines or papers, which can be filled with slanderous journalism.

We used to call this specific kind of writing, "yellow journalism" Apparently, it's fairly rewarding to make a tabloid filled with misinformation that is undependable and breathtaking tales, based upon manufacture. But some people today read the tales, and frequently replicate them as details. You could think, "It does not have any effect on fact, and individuals have a right for amusement, even if it's slanderous."

Think about this: All these very same men and women, who examine misinformation and think it, have as much right to vote within another election because you can. You will invest your own time exploring the truth, whilst somebody else, using an identical vote, bases their conclusions . That is the information age; however, it's likewise the corruption era.

What are a few "telltale" signs of tragedy? Whenever someone claims to be the manual to the sole path - see. This is a fantastic strategy for producing a"us against them" mindset. Exclusive and elitist classes have misinformed humankind long before yellowish journalism became increasingly popular.

As that applies to Yoga, politics, faith, doctrine and life - agreeing of speakers and governments who attempt to split. The ideal route for mankind to take would be modelled with loving-kindness. The results of an educated religious leader derive from tolerance, love, mercy, charity, empathy, and compassion.

NADA YOGA

A new fad now are Wisdom Schools. These are colleges include curricula according to learning how to employ the Wisdom Traditions and fundamental comprehension of cultures which were holistic in their own thinking. Science, faith, and the artwork have been intertwined in those schools, so you obtained confidential, esoteric understanding that wasn't just packed into the mind, but consumed by the entire body, the entire self. Considering that the Enlightenment, our foundation of knowledge was getting thinner. Material science is now all pervading into the stage that a number of us believe everything is created from matter and may be explained like that.

Quantum Physics in addition to theology, doctrine, and inherent understanding inform us of that this isn't correct. The Wisdom School differs from the ordinary institution now since it doesn't make individuals who may adhere to the program, or adhere to the information that they learned. They produce those who may create new info and provide new poses on the planet. I attended a few of those Wisdom Schools that's been in existence for many decades. This school educated on the basis of Creation Spirituality.

It created an effort to bring faith, science, as well as the arts back together back in something known as the Spiritual Warrior, and also the Warrior of Compassion. The Warrior of Compassion retrieved her capacity to say no or yes, to make choice when given the right info, and also to make a community in which it described what was delightful and desired rather than outsiders. Section of this job I do today, resulting in Sacred Union Ceremonies come as a consequence of attending this Wisdom School.

A huge portion of our service is composed of something named Nada Yoga, or the Yoga of Sound. Nada Yoga is a really ancient tradition which developed together with Yoga, such as Hatha Yoga, for the centuries. During the usage of this voice, musical ragas (climbs and tunes), and also the manipulation of this breath together with motion, Nada Yoga influences the nervous system. It contributes to a sense of calmness and relaxation and opens you to an experience with the Divine. It brings you into an area of calmness and stillness where you can actually listen to the noise of the world which is at the middle of our ancestors.

The Hindu faith, in addition to Yogic belief methods, Christianity as well as also the Abrahamic traditions always believed of this world as light, sound, and shaking. Through proper movement and salvation, and knowledge, an individual can align with the world and listen to the tune of the world and be one with it. An Individual may become, in other words, a person using all the Word of God or the Logos.

A lot of men and women in the west do not know a lot about Nada Yoga. Some people who consider themselves specialists in Hatha Yoga do not pay too much focus on it since they have not heard of it earlier. They believe that Nada Yoga is really singing devotional songs in Sanskrit. They frequently consider the historical heritage as a tool insincere and New Agey, and owing to their lack of religious development together with a lot of physical improvement due to performing Hatha Yoga, and they cannot differentiate what is really religious. The thing of Yoga is setting the self and stirring to the increased self. I believe this thought was abandoned by some of those men and women in the west since they've narrowed their perspective of Meditation into performing gymnastic feats, which may if one isn't cautious, harden the self rather than launch it.

Nada Yoga is a reintroduction of some other degree yoga to our society. Hatha is just 1 branch yoga from eight. Can it be any surprise that people in the west could embrace the maximum physical division as the sole branch? Additionally, there are seven additional branches and an unlimited number of forms chiefly since Yoga method to connect with God. That's that the God inside oneself and out of yourself. If you would like to go deeper in the practice, you do not necessarily have to devote up Hatha Yoga. It's strong and really good a hammering the self once done the correct way. What's essential is that you start to research more divisions and kinds of yoga, particularly Nada Yoga. It's straightforward and easy and it will if completed properly, connect you to a higher self so you will be alert and free of your negativity and projections which frequently drag us into depression, anger, nervousness and all the other drawbacks which are frequently the fruit of our youth at the west. Based on figures, nearly fifty percent of those taxpayers in the united states are currently on some kind of medicine for depression. This can be a indication that something's very, very incorrect.

KUNDALINI YOGA

The real source of Kundalini Yoga is headquartered at the mysticism of ancient India. With study, the link between the tradition of Kundalini Yoga and the philosophy of Kashmir Shaivism becomes apparent. Shiva himself is reputed to be the very first Guru from the Kundalini Yoga convention according to Kashmir Shaivism. Most historians concur that this particular practice of Yoga, that was made to elevate the Shakti power, relies upon the philosophical treatise of Patanjali known as the Yoga Sutras.

These sutras are thought to return to the second century BCE. Patanjali supplies us with an extremely systematic and scientific method of stirring and nourishing that the Kundalini energy. He also developed an eight-limbed method of Meditation that offers the adherent using moral, ethical, and physical instructions for getting and keeping a state of oneness with the Divine.

The early tantric doctrine of Kashmir Shaivism appeared in the eighth and seventh centuries BCE at Kashmir. In accordance with the convention, Shiva appeared in the kind of Srikanthanath to elucidate the holy knowledge that has been missing throughout the Kali Yuga or period of darkness.

Shiva's three-pronged trident is prepositive of those 3 facets of mysterious knowledge he educated: abheda, meaning presence without distinction, bhedabheda, presence together and without distinction, along with bheda or the adventure of presence as a distinguished being. These 3 countries of their experience of presence are all described in the scriptural texts, including that the TantrasBhairava, RudraTantras, along with the Shiva Tantras.

Kundalini was introduced into the West in 1969 from Yogi Bhajan. Yogi Bhajan has been a renowned master of Kundalini Yoga in India. After he travelled to the Westhe also introduced the practice of Kundalini Yoga into the mainstream as a integrated platform of religious expansion. He provided the mysterious practice of Kundalini Yoga, as a part, as a antidote into the maelstrom of drug misuse in the late night.

It's an excellent gift the esoteric understanding of Kundalini Yoga is now available to the West. A normal practice of Kundalini Yoga is believed to immediately influence human consciousness from the ability of the awakened Kundalini Shakti. Kundalinipractices concentrate specifically on the function of the remainder of the endocrine system onto an individual being's energy and well-being. The best objective of this sort of Yoga will be to ready the power method of a human being to maintain the ability of the awakened Kundalini Shakti. In time, could unite the awareness of this Yogi or Yogini into the awareness of God.

Most Yoga practices have parts of Kundalini Yoga inside them. There's a confusion regarding Kundalini and its link to novelty. Most newcomers to this practice are attracted to this by this attention , assuming the word, Kundalini Rising, describes a sort of climax. All Yoga provides the ideal of overall Enlightenment. YesKundalini Yoga is great for improving your sexual life, (as is Yoga), but let us analyze it a bit farther.

The meaning of Kundalini (in Sanskrit) could be

interpreted as acoiled, corporeal power' or unconscious, instinctive, libidinal force (Shakti)' that is located (curled upward) in the bottom of their spine. It's a religious energy or life force that's usually called a serpent. Thus the title - Kundalini (or even Kundala) -'what can be coiled, to spiral or to stunt'.Kundalini Yoga arouses this sleeping Kundalini Shakti (out of the coiled base)up the entire body, throughout the 6 chakras (travelling across the main stations of pranic energy from your system) to permeate the 7th chakra (the Crown), creating strength, personality, consciousness and consciousness. It's been known as'serpent power' and can be explained as NirmalaSrivastava as a'staying ability of pure appetite'. Describing the true location is quite hard, with a few stating it resides somewhere between the anus and the navel, but some say it's in the sacrum bone. Most of us believe this to some extent, particularly during prolonged intervals of excitement or danger - maybe together with the'flight or fight' adrenaline reaction.

Sexual is the most effective energy within your body - it must be to make life. Whenever some Yoga practices can impair sexual vitality, Kundalini Yoga adopts it and utilizes its own processes (asanas, meditations, passive and active kriya strings, command and pranayama) to channel sexual energy up the spine to enable spiritual improvement. To explain the first point made in this informative article - Kundalini Yoga is really excellent for changing ALL energies within the body, and this obviously contains sexual vitality. To notice, the most important objective of Kundalini Yoga isn't fantastic sex, but fantastic sex is a nice side effect of this.

Yogi Bhajan (who taught and practisedKundalini methods for at least 35 years) was clearly of the opinion that gender was sacred, ought to be earmarked for dedicated relationships and didn't urge casual sexual experiences in any way. Yogi Bhajan thought sacred sex had been gruesome love in actions with the two partners treating each other like holy temples of their celestial and his overpowering theme was -'Watch God in All'. He had been first to teach Kundalini Yoga publicly, touching many hearts, starting many heads and mentoring several politicians, statesmen and famous characters. He was equally at home if instruction at a boardroom or sitting on the grass in a park.

Kundalini Awakening Stages

Below are the phases that show the joys of Ida and Pingala (both left and right) and the fundamental station that flows throughout the chakras (SushumnaNadi - also referred to as the'silver cord'). These signify Kundalini Awakening in six phases;

Prana flowing in Ida or Pingala

Prana flowing in Ida and Pingala

Prana flowing in Sushumna

Kundalini energy awakens

Kundalini energy contributes upward

Kundalini climbs to Sahasrara (crown chakra)

Shakti and Shiva

The travel of Kundalini Yoga, resulting in Kundalini Awakening contributes to the understanding of the Complete at which consciousness divides itself into two elements which appear to be apart but can't exist without each other. They're known as Shiva (a stationary, formless quality) and Shakti (a lively, creative part of understanding). They are sometimes conceptualized as deities or principles / procedures of the world. In any event, the travel is an internal one travelling to the centre of someone's own consciousness. Interestingly enough, a few individuals have undergone spontaneous Kundalini Awakening without performing any deliberate practices.

After Kundalini Awakening has happened, also becomes even established during meditation, Kundalini was proven to mechanically purify the human body and dispel all psychological, bodily and spiritual clutter. Planning for Kundalini Awakening is quite important since when it happens, there's a particular quantity of effort and time required to combine the facets to the human body and character. But after real Enlightenment and also Self-Realization, the entire body grows more energetic and zestful, the face younger and also the character magnetic and beautiful.

CONCLUSION

These Yoga meditation techniques have been used for centuries for spiritual purposes. However, they can also be used as natural pain relief methods. By applying the meditation techniques specifically for pain control, practitioners are able to have a positive effect on such severe kinds of pain.

Please be aware that, while yoga has a spiritual part, it's not a religion. You don't need to believe in any specific deity or even to believe in God at all to practice yoga. People of all faiths, as well as agnostics and atheists, are regular yoga practitioners. And it's fine to embrace those aspects of the practice that appeal to you and ignore the rest. Modifying the practice to suit your needs applies not just to postures but to the spiritual dimension as well.